Facial Scar Management

Editor

DAVID B. HOM

FACIAL PLASTIC SURGERY
CLINICS OF NORTH AMERICA

www.facialplastic.theclinics.com

Consulting Editor
J. REGAN THOMAS

February 2017 • Volume 25 • Number 1

ELSEVIER

1600 John F. Kennedy Boulevard • Suite 1800 • Philadelphia, Pennsylvania, 19103-2899

http://www.theclinics.com

FACIAL PLASTIC SURGERY CLINICS OF NORTH AMERICA Volume 25, Number 1
February 2017 ISSN 1064-7406, ISBN-13: 978-0-323-49647-6

Editor: Jessica McCool
Developmental Editor: Alison Swety

Facial Plastic Surgery Clinics of North America (ISSN 1064-7406) is published quarterly by Elsevier Inc., 360 Park Avenue South, New York, NY 10010-1710. Months of issue are February, May, August, and November. Business and Editorial Offices: 1600 John F. Kennedy Blvd., Suite 1800, Philadelphia, PA 19103-2899. Periodicals postage paid at New York, NY, and additional mailing offices. Subscription prices are $390.00 per year (US individuals), $592.00 per year (US institutions), $445.00 per year (Canadian individuals), $737.00 per year (Canadian institutions), $535.00 per year (foreign individuals), $737.00 per year (foreign institutions), $100.00 per year (US students), and $255.00 per year (foreign students). Foreign air speed delivery is included in all *Clinics* subscription prices. All prices are subject to change without notice. POSTMASTER: Send address changes to *Facial Plastic Surgery Clinics*, Elsevier Health Sciences Division, Subscription Customer Service, 3251 Riverport Lane, Maryland Heights, MO 63043. **Customer service: 1-800-654-2452 (US and Canada); 1-314-447-8871 (outside US and Canada); Fax: 314-447-8029; E-mail: journalscustomerservice-usa@elsevier.com (for print support); journalsonline support-usa@elsevier.com (for online support).**

Reprints. For copies of 100 or more of articles in this publication, please contact the Commercial Reprints Department, Elsevier Inc., 360 Park Avenue South, New York, NY 10010-1710. Tel.: 212-633-3874; Fax: 212-633-3820; E-mail: reprints@elsevier.com.

Facial Plastic Surgery Clinics of North America is covered in *MEDLINE/PubMed* (*Index Medicus*).

Contributors

CONSULTING EDITOR

J. REGAN THOMAS, MD, FACS
Professor and Chairman, Department of
Otolaryngology, University of Illinois at
Chicago, Chicago, Illinois

EDITOR

DAVID B. HOM, MD, FACS
Professor and Director, Division of Facial
Plastic and Reconstructive Surgery,
Departments of Otolaryngology – Head & Neck
Surgery and Dermatology, University of
Cincinnati College of Medicine, Cincinnati
Children's Hospital Medical Center, Cincinnati,
Ohio

AUTHORS

CHRISTIAN BARNES, MD
UC Irvine Department of Head & Neck Surgery,
Orange, California

KOFI DEREK BOAHENE, MD
Associate Professor, Department of
Otorhinolaryngology, The Johns Hopkins
Hospital, Baltimore, Maryland

LUCAS M. BRYANT, MD
Resident Physician, Department of
Otolaryngology – Head & Neck Surgery,
Thomas Jefferson University Hospital, Thomas
Jefferson University, Philadelphia,
Pennsylvania

BENJAMIN P. CAUGHLIN, MD
Clinical Instructor, UC Irvine Department of
Head & Neck Surgery, Orange, California;
Facial Plastic and Reconstructive Surgery,
Chicago, Illinois

CHRISTOPHER B. CHAMBERS, MD
Assistant Professor, Division of Oculoplastic
Surgery, Department of Ophthalmology,
University of Washington School of Medicine,
Seattle, Washington

ERIK WILLIAM EVANS, DDS, MD
Assistant Professor of Surgery, Division of Oral
and Maxillofacial Surgery, University of
Cincinnati Medical Center, Veterans Affairs
Medical Center, Cincinnati Children's Hospital
Medical Center, Cincinnati, Ohio

FRED G. FEDOK, MD, FACS
Adjunct Professor, Department of Surgery,
USA Medical Center, The University of South
Alabama, Mobile, Alabama; Fedok Plastic
Surgery, Foley, Alabama; Facial Plastic and
Reconstructive Surgery, Penn State Hershey
Medical Center, Hershey, Pennsylvania

RICHARD D. GENTILE, MD, MBA
Gentile Facial Plastic & Aesthetic Laser Center,
Boardman, Ohio

RYAN HEFFELFINGER, MD
Assistant Professor, Division of Facial Plastic &
Reconstructive Surgery, Department of
Otolaryngology – Head & Neck Surgery,
Thomas Jefferson University Hospital, Thomas
Jefferson University, Philadelphia,
Pennsylvania

DAVID B. HOM, MD, FACS
Professor and Director, Division of Facial Plastic and Reconstructive Surgery, Departments of Otolaryngology – Head & Neck Surgery and Dermatology, University of Cincinnati College of Medicine, Cincinnati Children's Hospital Medical Center, Cincinnati, Ohio

JOHN KIM
Kaiser Permanente, Southern California, Riverside, California

JESSYKA G. LIGHTHALL, MD
Assistant Professor, Division of Otolaryngology – Head & Neck Surgery, Director, Facial Plastic and Reconstructive Surgery, Penn State Hershey Medical Center, Hershey, Pennsylvania

KRISTEN S. MOE, MD
Professor and Chief, Division of Facial Plastic and Reconstructive Surgery, Departments of Otolaryngology and Neurological Surgery, University of Washington School of Medicine, Seattle, Washington

J. STUART NELSON, MD, PhD
UC Irvine Department of Head & Neck Surgery, Orange, California

JAMES A. OWUSU, MD
Assistant Professor, Department of Otorhinolaryngology – Head and Neck Surgery, University of Texas Health Sciences Center at Houston, Houston, Texas

BHARAT PANUGANTI, MD
Resident Surgeon, Division of Otolaryngology – Head and Neck Surgery, University of California, San Diego, San Diego, California

ASHLEY RUDNICK, BS
Miami, Florida

AKSHAY SANAN, MD
Resident Physician, Department of Otolaryngology – Head & Neck Surgery, Thomas Jefferson University Hospital, Thomas Jefferson University, Philadelphia, Pennsylvania

MARTY O. VISSCHER, PhD
Skin Sciences Program, Cincinnati, Ohio

JILL S. WAIBEL, MD
Board Certified Dermatologist, Private Practice, Miami Dermatology and Laser Institute, Subsection Chief of Dermatology, Baptist Hospital, Voluntary Assistant Professor, Dermatology Faculty, Miller School of Medicine, University of Miami, Miami, Florida

DEBORAH WATSON, MD, FACS
Professor of Surgery, Division of Otolaryngology – Head and Neck Surgery, University of California, San Diego, San Diego, California

JAMIE L. WELSHHANS, MD
Division of Facial Plastic and Reconstructive Surgery, Department of Otolaryngology – Head & Neck Surgery, University of Cincinnati College of Medicine, Cincinnati Children's Hospital Medical Center, Cincinnati, Ohio

BRIAN J.F. WONG, MD, PhD
UC Irvine Department of Head & Neck Surgery, Orange, California

Contents

anatomy of nasal subunits and their underlying structural framework limit surgical options in nasal scar revision compared with other areas of the face. An understanding of a variety of laser technologies and their specific applications can vastly aid in fine, controlled scar revision. Achieving optimal scar reduction regularly requires multiple stages of intervention, close follow-up, and repeat procedures.

Lip and chin scarring occurs owing to reconstruction of congenital, cancer resection, or traumatic defects. Knowledge of lip anatomy and function is critical to optimize results. Realistic expectations should be established before intervention. Scar revision and reconstruction is ideally performed with a subunit approach, placing scars along aesthetic borders and performing subunit reconstruction to camouflage scars. Surgical techniques include direct excision, scar reorientation, local flap rearrangement, pedicled flaps, and regional or free flaps. Resurfacing/adjunctive procedures play important roles in the treatment of scars. This article reviews the anatomy, patient assessment, and techniques used in scar revision of the perioral region.

This article provides a review of the surgical and nonsurgical options available to manage a variety of auricular scars. The basics of wound healing are discussed in addition to the etiology of keloids and the cauliflower ear. Many auricular scars can be revised with scar excision techniques, but separate discussions for the treatment of keloids and the cauliflower ear are provided. The management plan for auricular scarring requires appropriate patient counseling regarding the risk of recurrence in keloids, regrowth of scar tissue in cauliflower ears, scar hypertrophy at the line of closure, widening of the scar, and persisting ear contour deformities.

The scalp presents many challenges to the reconstructive surgeon given its visible nature and the various considerations that must be given for optimal reconstruction. In this article, we review the anatomy of the scalp, the various options for reconstruction, and important considerations for improving the chances of optimal reconstruction of scalp defects.

Mucosal wounds tend to heal more rapidly than skin wounds and with minimal to no scar formation and hence have a minimal impact on function or aesthetics. This is likely due to differences in the magnitude and timing of the various factors that contribute to wound healing. Some examples of these differences are fibroblast proliferation, transforming growth factor-β, macrophages, neutrophils, and T cells. Other factors, such as the moist environment, contribute to the favorable wound-healing characteristics of mucosa.

Scarring of the neck affects millions of people every year. The appearance of neck scarring can be disturbing both physically and psychologically. Scarring of the neck can be accompanied by morbidities because of the limitation of functional motion of the neck. Treatment options and modalities for reduction and prevention of scar formation include topical steroids, intralesional steroids, interferon, 5-fluorouracil, silicone gel, radiation, laser therapy, and surgeries. There is no general consensus in the literature as to the optimal treatment of neck scarring. Patients should understand that the scar is likely to be improved but not eliminated by treatment.

Contemporary Topics Relevant to Facial Scarring

Treatment of facial scars is a multispecialty endeavor for optimal patient recovery. One new innovation helping in facial scar treatments are lasers. Fractional laser predictably (tunable) disrupts the barrier of the skin creating deep channels that allow the delivery of drug and cellular materials; this is called laser-assisted drug delivery (LAD). Without exception thus far, LAD has been found to enhance the local uptake of any drug or substance applied to the skin. These zones may be used postoperatively to deliver drugs and other substances to create an enhanced scar therapeutic response to drug or substance applied to the skin.

Skin coloration is highly diverse, partly due to the presence of pigmentation. Color variation is related to the extent of ultraviolet radiation exposure, as well as other factors. Inherent skin coloration arises from differences in basal epidermal melanin amount and type. Skin color is influenced by both the quantity and distribution of melanocytes. The effectiveness of inherent pigmentation for protecting living cells also varies. This article discusses skin color, pigmentation, and ethnicity in relation to clinical practice. Color perception, skin typing/classification, and quantitation of pigmentation are reviewed in relation to ethnicity, environmental stresses/irritants, and potential treatment effects.

FACIAL PLASTIC SURGERY CLINICS OF NORTH AMERICA

THE CLINICS ARE AVAILABLE ONLINE!
Access your subscription at:
www.theclinics.com

Preface

Facial Scar Management

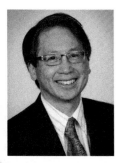

David B. Hom, MD, FACS
Editor

Cutaneous scarring is an inevitable consequence following surgery and deeper dermal injuries. Scars on the face can be especially disconcerting to patients due to their public visibility. Facial scars also can give significant morbidity, ranging from functional problems impairing eating, speaking, nasal breathing, and eyelid closure, which can result in long-lasting psychological impairment.

Important principles and management techniques can be employed that can minimize scarring to improve both patient functional outcomes and satisfaction.

Many scar references describe how to manage scars by using numerous techniques using a generic perspective. However, another conceptual approach to manage scars is categorizing them by anatomic facial site (**Fig. 1**).

Classifying scars by facial subunits (forehead, periorbital region, cheeks, nose, perioral/chin region, auricle, scalp, neck) can be helpful because each region has distinct skin properties. Specifically, facial skin within each facial subunit can have different dermal thicknesses, elasticity, and vascularity with dissimilar underlying subcutaneous tissue and bone. Thus, scar formation can result in different physical sequelae at each of the various facial regions. Therefore, the management of a scar can be region specific due to these properties.

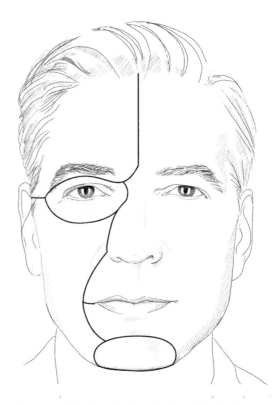

Fig. 1. Facial subunits for which articles in this issue are subdivided.

Facial Plast Surg Clin N Am 25 (2017) ix–x
http://dx.doi.org/10.1016/j.fsc.2016.10.001
1064-7406/17/© 2016 Published by Elsevier Inc.

This issue of *Facial Plastic Surgery Clinics of North America* specifically approaches scar management according to the various topographic facial regions. In the first section, "Treating Scars in Relation to Facial Regions," the first article highlights general concepts to minimize scarring followed by scar principles for each facial aesthetic unit relevant to that specific anatomic site. In addition, a fascinating article about the unique properties of oral cavity scarring is included, which is quite distinct from skin scarring.

In the second section, "Contemporary Topics Relevant to Facial Scarring," additional contemporary topics relevant to scarring are presented. This includes the use of lasers as a means of drug delivery to treat scarring and the current status of ethnic pigmentation in relation to scarring.

It has been a pleasure to be a guest editor for this topic on scars that we all encounter with our patients. I hope this issue will be very informative to you, as it has been for me, in approaching patients with scars.

I would like to sincerely thank the article authors for their diligence and significant contributions to this issue of *Facial Plastic Surgery Clinics of North America*.

David B. Hom, MD, FACS
Division of Facial Plastic and
Reconstructive Surgery
Departments of Otolaryngology –
Head and Neck Surgery and Dermatology
University of Cincinnati College of Medicine
Cincinnati Children's Hospital Medical Center
PO Box 670528
231 Albert Sabin Way
Cincinnati, OH 45267-0528, USA

E-mail address:
david.hom@uc.edu

Treating Scars in Relation to Facial Regions

Soft Tissue Principles to Minimize Scarring
An Overview

Jamie L. Welshhans, MD[a], David B. Hom, MD, FACS[b,c],*

KEYWORDS

- Scar • Scarring • Scar treatment • Scar revision • Ointment • Silicone • Laser • Dermabrasion

KEY POINTS

- Patient factors include skin type, medical conditions, ethnicity, medications, and soft tissue healing. Patient perception plays a role in the scar result.
- Preoperative planning, intraoperative tissue handling, and suture techniques are vitally important to optimize wound healing and minimize scarring.
- Postoperative use of ointments, taping, silicone, and sun protective products as well as adjunctive procedures (dermabrasion, scar revision, and laser therapy) can assist in the final overall scar appearance.

INTRODUCTION

Scarring is an inevitable consequence of surgery. Facial scars, due to their public visibility, can be very disconcerting to patients. They can have significant morbidity, ranging from functional problems to psychological sequela.[1] Important principles and management techniques can be used that can minimize scarring to improve both patient functional outcome and satisfaction. The purpose of this article is to give a broad and practical overview of clinical measures to reduce facial scarring.

SCARRING IN RELATION TO WOUND HEALING

Scars form when the deep reticular layer of the dermis is violated. As a part of the healing process, the body forms new collagen fibers resulting in a scar. Four phases of wound healing occur following a surgical incision. They are coagulation and hemostasis, inflammation, proliferation, and remodeling. A scar is formed primarily during the latter 2 phases. During proliferation, fibroblasts migrate into the wound to begin the process of making new collagen, which will eventually become a scar. New collagen is primarily type III collagen and is replaced with type I over time. As the scar gets stronger with time, wound strength approaches 70% of its original strength at 6 weeks but will never surpass 80% of its original skin strength. Remodeling is the last stage of wound healing in conjunction with contraction, which may last as long as 1 to 2 years.

Neither Dr D.B. Hom nor Dr J.L. Welshhans have anything to disclose.
[a] Division of Facial Plastic and Reconstructive Surgery, Department of Otolaryngology-Head & Neck Surgery, Cincinnati Children's Hospital Medical Center, University of Cincinnati College of Medicine, Cincinnati, OH, USA; [b] Division of Facial Plastic and Reconstructive Surgery, Department of Otolaryngology-Head & Neck Surgery, University of Cincinnati College of Medicine, PO Box 670528, 231 Albert Sabin Way, Cincinnati, OH 45267-0528, USA; [c] Department of Dermatology, Cincinnati Children's Hospital Medical Center, University of Cincinnati College of Medicine, PO Box 670528, 231 Albert Sabin Way, Cincinnati, OH 45267-0528, USA
* Corresponding author. Division of Facial Plastic and Reconstructive Surgery, Department of Otolaryngology-Head & Neck Surgery, University of Cincinnati College of Medicine, PO Box 670528, 231 Albert Sabin Way, Cincinnati, OH 45267-0528.
E-mail address: david.hom@uc.edu

Facial Plast Surg Clin N Am 25 (2017) 1–13
http://dx.doi.org/10.1016/j.fsc.2016.08.002

Within the extracellular matrix, the fibrin-rich matrix during the inflammatory phase transforms to a collagen-rich extracellular matrix during the proliferative phase. During the remodeling phase, collagen deposition and cross-linking occur, forming an organized collagen fiber network, which later undergoes wound contraction as fibroblasts transform into myofibroblast. The collagen breakdown is controlled by matrix metalloproteinases.[2] In addition, dermal extracellular matrix transformation occurs with fibronectin followed by hyaluronan (4–6 days) and then with proteoglycans deposition (7–10 days).

Any factors that delay wound healing will increase risk for scarring. Thus, measures to optimize dermal wound healing will result in reduced scar formation. Factors to ensure proper wound healing include (1) adequate nutrition, (2) sufficient blood supply, (3) proper wound management, (4) wound pressure relief, and (5) minimizing bacterial contamination.

RELEVANT ANATOMY
Skin Structure and Skin Condition

The skin consists of several layers: epidermis, papillary dermis reticular dermis, and hypodermis (**Fig. 1**). The adnexal structures in the dermis (ie, hair follicles, apocrine and ermine glands) serve as progenitor cell sources for epithelialization.[3] When injury occurs in the deep reticular layer of the dermis that is allowed to heal by secondary intention, more scarring usually occurs. Incisions through thicker skin tend to scar more than thin skin. Especially in thick sebaceous skin, incisions tend to scar easier.

FACIAL AREAS PRONE TO SCARRING

Convex surfaces of the face, such as the chin, cheek, forehead, and nasal tip, are more prone to hypertrophic, widened scars compared with other regions of the face.

Also, areas in close proximity to mobile regions of the face have an increased risk to have widened scars due to the continuous pull on the incision. In this instance, taping the incision for several months after suture is removed may help reduce pulling on the incision as it matures, resulting in a less widened scar.

PATIENT FACTORS
Medical Conditions

Several medical conditions and medications can predispose a surgical patient to scarring (**Box 1**). Patients with hyperplastic joints have increased elastin in the dermis and are more prone to scarring.[4] Surgeons should consider checking for signs of hyperelasticity by asking the patient to bend his thumb to his forearm or to touch his tongue to his nose (**Fig. 2**). An additional patient factor that can contribute to scarring is age. In younger patients, the remodeling phase of the scar is more prolonged, resulting in increased erythema and hypertrophy. Remodeling becomes more adultlike after puberty.[4] Any condition that increases the propensity for a prolonged inflammatory reaction during wound healing, such as an infection or a foreign body reaction, increases the probability of more scarring. Other medical problems, such as diabetes, collagen vascular disease, hypothyroidism, immunocompromised states, and diseases with delayed healing, have an increased risk for scarring.

Patients with poor nutritional status who have decreased wound healing are more prone to scar. Specific nutritional deficiencies known to delay healing are vitamin C deficiency, which is necessary for the hydroxylation of lysine and proline for collagen cross-linking. Zinc and copper are also required for collagen cross-linking, and vitamin K is necessary for clotting and prothrombin production. As a result, deficiencies in these vitamins impede healing.

Patients with a history of previous radiation have poor wound healing and scarring. Radiation affects wound healing by causing obliterative endarteritis, excessive fibrosis, and an aberration of normal cellular replication. A total radiation dose greater than 50 Gy is consistently associated with poor wound healing.[5] Patients who smoke are also more likely to heal poorly and have a higher risk for scarring due to the vasoconstrictive effects of nicotine. Medications, such as corticosteroids and chemotherapy agents, also slow down healing and increase risk for scarring.

Type of Skin Injury

Planned, sterile surgical wounds will have less scarring compared with traumatic wounds. Traumatic wounds heal with more scarring due to a heightened inflammatory response from foreign bodies and bacteria inoculation. Infected wounds ($>10^5$ microorganisms per gram of tissue) induce a longer inflammatory phase of wound healing, and therefore, heal with more scarring. In addition, burn-inflicted trauma is more likely to result in scar hypertrophy.

Topographically, scars can be classified into several types, as seen in **Fig. 3**. Linear wounds that are perpendicular to the relaxed skin tension line (RSTL) make scars more apparent.[4]

Ethnicity

Ethnicity plays a role in scar formation. Patients with Fitzpatrick skin types IVtoVI are at increased

A

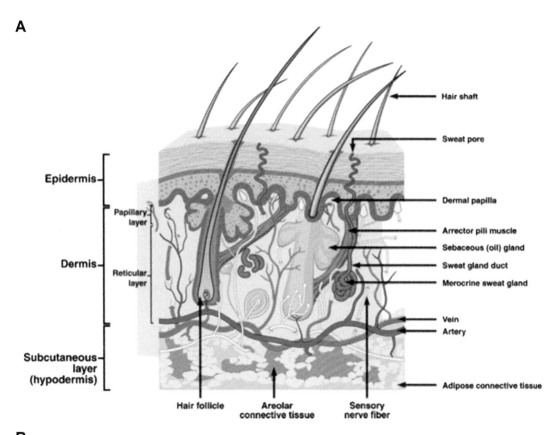

Epidermis

Papillary layer

Dermis

Reticular layer

Subcutaneous layer (hypodermis)

Hair shaft

Sweat pore

Dermal papilla

Arrector pili muscle

Sebaceous (oil) gland

Sweat gland duct

Merocrine sweat gland

Vein

Artery

Adipose connective tissue

Hair follicle   Areolar connective tissue   Sensory nerve fiber

B

NORMAL SKIN

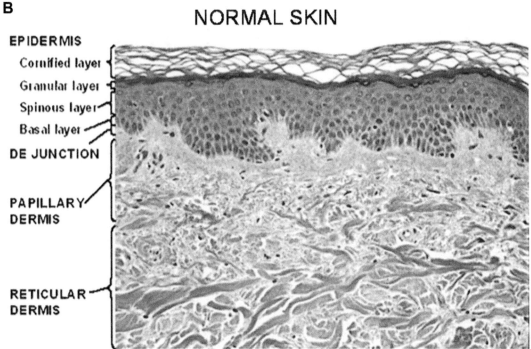

EPIDERMIS
Cornified layer
Granular layer
Spinous layer
Basal layer
DE JUNCTION

PAPILLARY DERMIS

RETICULAR DERMIS

Fig. 1. Skin anatomy. Diagram (*A*) and histological section (*B*) showing the layers of human skin. (*From* Hebda PA. Skin wound healing. In: Hom DB, Hebda PA, Gosain AK, et al, editors. Essential tissue healing of the face and neck. Shelton, CT: People's Medical Publishing House; 2009; with permission.)

risk for scar hypertrophy, hyperpigmentation, and hypopigmentation. Specifically, Asians have an increased propensity for hyperpigmentation and widened scars. In addition, African American patients and those of other races with darker complexion (ie, Hispanic, Asian Indian) are more likely to have hypertrophic scar formation.[6]

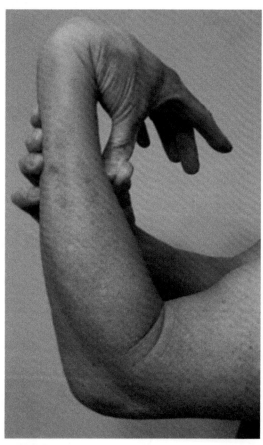

Fig. 2. Hyperelasticity. A patient who can bend his thumb to his forearm as shown in the photo has joint hyperelasticity, which gives an increased propensity for scarring.

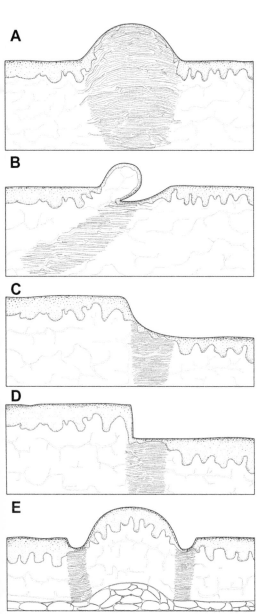

Fig. 3. Scar types. (*A*) Keloid or hypertrophic scar lacking adnexal structures with thin epidermis. (*B*) Oblique scar in dermal depth with slanted contraction. (*C*) Uneven sloping scar with various dermal depths. (*D*) Iatrogenic step off scar from inaccurate apposition of skin edges. (*E*) Trap Coro or pin cushioning scar from circumferential contraction. (*Adapted from* Rosie T, Harahap M. Scar Analysis and treatment selection: the "geo-topographic approach." In: Harahap M, editor. Surgical techniques for cutaneous scar revision. New York: Marcel Dekker; 2000. p. 81.)

AGE

Children can be more vulnerable to dermal scarring because the remodeling phase of healing is more prolonged than adults, resulting in increased scar erythema and scar hypertrophy. Thus, some think that elective cosmetic scar revision in children should be delayed until puberty unless a functional deficit is occurring.[7]

PRETREATMENT OF TISSUE BEFORE SURGERY

Very little is described in the literature about pretreating tissue before a surgical procedure. Optimizing the preoperative wound healing state is essential (**Box 2**). These important common factors include maximizing the nutritional status, controlling diabetes, and reducing smoking. In fact, any component that delays healing increases the risk for scarring. If a patient has been taking isotretinoin (Accutane), elective skin ablative procedures requiring re-epithelialization (such as laser ablative resurfacing, dermabrasion, chemical peel) should be avoided for at least 1 year. This recommendation is because isotretinoins cause sebaceous gland atrophy, which diminishes an important epithelial cell source. When a partial thickness wound does not re-epithelialize within 3 weeks, scarring significantly increases if one is suspicious for a higher risk of scarring before a skin ablative procedure. A test dose can be delivered behind the ear to determine the pigmentary and scar skin response.

Efforts should be made to minimize dermal inflammation during the acute phase of skin healing. This belief is because if a wound remains persistently inflamed longer than 3 weeks, from a foreign body reaction or dermal infection, long-term scarring significantly increases.

A patient with a history of fever blisters should take prophylactic antiviral medications (ie, valacyclovir) before during and after a skin ablative procedure to avoid a herpetic outbreak periorally, thus increasing the risks of scarring from these healing vesicles.

MINIMIZING FUTURE SCARRING DURING A PROCEDURE WITH PLANNED INCISIONS

The facial subunits consist of major aesthetic units comprising the forehead, eyes, nose, perioral region, chin, and cheek (**Fig. 4**). Facial aesthetic units and subunits are visual anatomic boundaries. Light reflection and shadows help conceal scars along these facial aesthetic borders. These aesthetic units can be subdivided into additional anatomic subunits. For example, the nose can be divided into nasal tip, dorsum, columella, soft tissue triangles, sidewalls, and nasal alar regions. Planned incisions along these aesthetic facial structures assist in camouflaging the scar. Scars

Box 2
Practical guidelines for optimal wound healing to minimize scarring

- Debride necrotic tissue to decrease infection risk.
- Maintain fresh wound edges along the incision to encourage epithelialization.
- Irrigate copiously to clean the wound and remove foreign bodies. Irrigation can be performed with normal saline or commercial wound cleanser. Irrigation is the single most effective technique to accomplish wound cleaning.
- Obtain hemostasis and place drains to prevent any excess fluid collection (ie, hematoma, seroma) and to avoid infection.
- Absorb excess wound exudate to prevent maceration of surrounding skin.
- Divert any salivary drainage away from the wound to minimize bacterial contamination.
- Maintain a moist wound environment with topical ointments or hydrogels to encourage epithelialization.
- Protect the wound from trauma.
- In wounds with potential for infection, institute appropriate oral and topical antibiotics for 7 to 10 days. Abrasions and wounds can be covered with hydrogel sheeting for exudative wounds or clear transparent dressing (ie, Tegaderm, Opposite) for nonexudative wounds.
- To avoid cellular damage, do not repetitively apply skin cleansers (ie, hydrogen peroxide, Betadine, Hibiclens) in a wound.

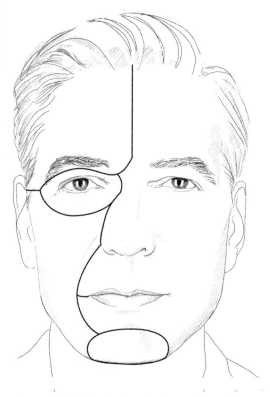

Fig. 4. Facial subunits for which articles in this issue are subdivided.

from incisions are more concealed when the incision is within the RSTL, along the facial subunit boundaries, within a hair-bearing area, or within orifices.

To minimize trap door scar defects, it is preferable to create incisions with straight lines and angles rather than circular incisions. These circular wounds are often created by Mohs micrographic surgery. In these cases, a small amount of additional tissue can be removed to transform the circular defect into a rhombic shape for skin flap repair, reducing the risk for a trap door deformity.

Minimizing soft tissue trauma is essential in creating the best possible postoperative outcome. Using the most appropriate instrumentation for each region of the face is important, as described in the other articles of this issue. Using small, toothed atraumatic forceps (ie, 0.5 mm or Bishops) or small Guthrie skin hooks when closing the skin helps avoid epidermal crushing. Furthermore, grabbing the dermis rather than the epidermis during wound closure prevents epidermal injury that can lead to scarring in some cases. In addition, to avoid burn injury to the skin, a protected tip unipolar bovine cautery or protected bipolar forceps cautery should be used for precise hemostasis.

When repairing a defect with a skin graft, wound contraction plays a major role in scarring. Full-thickness skin grafts that contract less than split-thickness grafts should be used at facial sites that are vulnerable to further wound contraction, giving functional deficits (such as the mobile tissue regions of the face: eyelid, brow, nostrils, and perioral region).

Suture Technique

The first aspect of suture technique is choosing the most appropriate suture. Buried sutures should be absorbable and serve as the anchor to keep the dermal edges together so that minimal tension is needed for the skin surface sutures. **Table 1** lists absorbable sutures available with their physical properties. The authors prefer to use Poliglecaprone (Monocryl) and Polygactin 910 (Vicryl) sutures for buried interrupted anchor sutures. Vicryl is a strong absorbable polyfilament suture, which has 50% tensile strength at 21 days and lacks suture memory, thus making it easy to work with. However, Vicryl can also elicit an inflammatory dermal reaction. Monocryl is a monofilament absorbable suture having more suture memory than Vicryl. It has 40% tensile strength at 14 days. Other common anchor suture choices include polydioxanone (PDSII), which has 25% tensile strength at 42 days. This monofilament suture gives a longer incisional strength duration for an anticipated slower healing wound. Surface skin sutures are placed not tightly in a simple, interrupted, running or intracuticular fashion to re-approximate the skin edges. Vertical mattress sutures can be placed to ensure skin eversion of the skin edges. The skin surface closure should have no tension. If the deeper layer is not well approximated, scar widening will occur. A preferred suture choice for cosmetic closure is Prolene or nylon suture because it is least reactive. Sutures should be removed in a timely manner to avoid persistent scar tracking from the suture entry and exit holes. If one plans to have the skin surface sutures remain longer and to avoid the "railroad tracking" appearance, a running intracuticular closure is beneficial. Another consideration would be to use a quick absorbing suture (ie, fast gut, plain gut, or mild chromic suture), which spontaneously breaks within 7 days. This suture is a good choice in children when suture removal is difficult.

The second aspect is properly passing of the suture through the dermal tissue. The needle should enter and exit the skin at the same dermal depth level on each side to realign the skin surfaces (**Fig. 5**). It is important for scar outcomes that the skin edges are slightly everted during closure. The skin edges should not be inverted, uneven, or under any tension.

Surgical Choices for Scar Revision

Managing patient expectations in scar revision

When it comes to revising a surgical scar, some patients may have unrealistic expectations because they expect the scar to totally disappear. It is imperative to inform patients of realistic scar revision goals and objectives that can be achieved. It is also important to determine from the patient what their top priority is for scar treatment. Is the goal to improve its raised appearance, width, color, tightness, texture, length, orientation, or location? By discussing realistic goals that can be achieved beforehand, the patient will more likely be satisfied with their scar revision.

Especially with a history of hypertrophic scars or a higher Fitzpatrick types (IV to VI), the patient should be warned that a higher risk of scarring and pigmentation exists. To help determine this risk, prior healed lacerations and incisions could be examined to see how the patient scarred in the past.

Box 3 summarizes scar revision modalities. A brief highlight of some basic surgical scar revision principles follows in later discussion. Ideally, when designing a scar, the linear incision should be parallel within the RSTL for the best cosmetic result.[8]

A very useful technique to change the direction of a scar is performing a Z-plasty. In addition to changing the direction the scar to allow it to fall more in the RSTLs or along facial unit boundaries, a Z-plasty can be used to (1) lengthen the scar to prevent surrounding contraction, (2) flatten a scar over an uneven surface, and (3) break up a long scar into smaller ones (**Fig. 6**).

The general principle of the Z-plasty consists of a central limb with 2 parallel lateral limbs that arise from the central limb. All limbs are the same length, and the lateral limbs form an equivalent angle ranging from 30° to 60° with respect to the central limb.[9] The flaps are then lifted as 2 triangles and then transposed. Clinically, the authors think that the 60° angle is most useful, which can lengthen the central limb of the scar by 75% (**Fig. 7**).

A W-plasty is also useful in breaking up a longitudinal scar into a smaller one. However, it does not lengthen the scar or release scar contracture along the central limb of the scar. A W-plasty is most useful on the cheek and forehead. The apex angles of the zigzag pattern of a W-plasty should be 45° to 80° (**Fig. 8**).

If the scar is longer (>4 cm), a geometric broken line closure is more appropriate because it removes the regularity of a W-plasty for longer lengths. Geometric broken line closure combines geometric shapes including triangles, rectangles,

Table 1
Properties of commonly used absorbable sutures

Suture	Configuration	Tensile Strength	Knot Tying	Knot Security	Tissue Reaction	Absorption Time	Uses
Surgical gut (plain gut or catgut)	Twisted	Poor at 7–10 d	Fair	Poor	Significant	6–8 wk	Subcutaneous
Surgical fast-absorbing gut	Twisted	0 at 7 d	Fair	Poor	Moderate	3–6 wk	Epidermis
Surgical chromic gut	Twisted	Poor at 21–23 d	Poor	Poor	Moderate	8–10 wk	Subcutaneous, oral tongue, or mucosa
Polygactin 910 (Vicryl)	Braided	75% at 14 d, 50% at 21 d, 5% at 30 d	Good	Good	Low	8–10 wk	Subcutaneous, fascia, vessel ligature
Vicryl Rapide	Braided	50% at 5 d, 0 at 14 d	Good	Good	Low	6 wk	Mucosa, epidermis
Polyglycolic acid (Dexon)	Braided	50% at 21 d	Good	Good	Low	7–14 wk	Subcutaneous, vessel ligature
PDSII	Monofilament	70% at 14 d, 50% at 28 d, 25% at 42 d	Fair	Good	Low	24–46 wk	Subcutaneous (high-tension areas), contaminated tissue
Polyglyconate (Maxon)	Monofilament	70% at 14 d, 55% at 21 d	Fair	Good	Low	26 wk	Subcutaneous, vessel ligature at high tension
Poliglecaprone (Monocryl)	Monofilament	6%–70% at 7 d, 30%–40% at 14 d	Good	Good	Low	13–17 wk skin closure	Subcuticular
Panaryl braided synthetic	Braided	90% at 6 wk, 80% at 3 mo	Good	Low	Low	18+ mo	Extremity closure

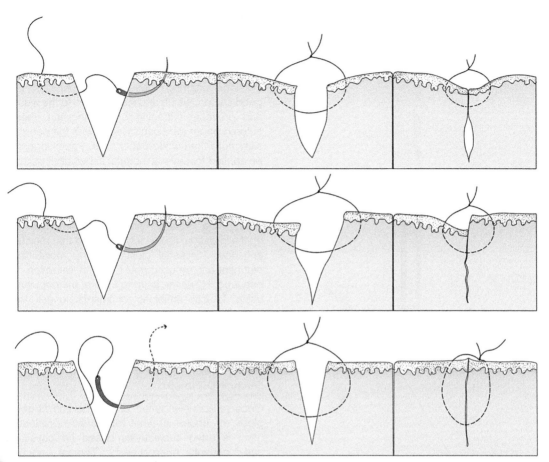

Fig. 5. Skin edge approximation with sutures. Top row: surface sutures are placed too superficial in depth leaving deeper empty space, which will contract and cause indented scar. Middle row: surface sutures are placed at uneven depths resulting in step off. Bottom row: the optimal suture approximation with similar suture depths.

Box 3
Scar revision modalities

1. Surgical scar revision methods
   a. Fusiform scar excision and serial excision
   b. Breaking up the scar: Z-plasty, W-plasty, geometric broken line
   c. Punch excision
   d. Skin grafting: punch excision and graft replacement
   e. Excision with skin flap or graft coverage
   f. Dermabrasion
   g. Laser (CO_2 or Nd:YAG)
   h. Tissue augmentation (dermis, fat, fascia)
2. Minimally invasive methods
   a. Injectable dermal augmentation fillers (autogenous, allogeneic, synthetic)
   b. Silicone gel sheeting or gel
   c. Physical modalities: compression, irradiation, cryoinjury
   d. Pharmaceutical medications: steroids, fibroblast, and collagen synthesis or cross-linking inhibitors, immune modulators

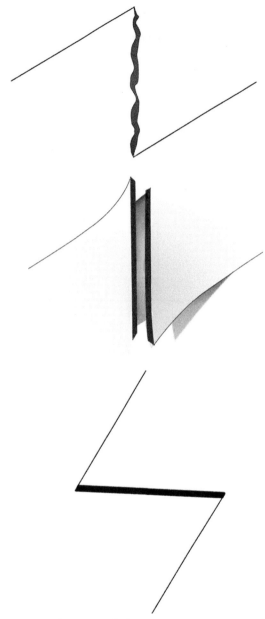

Fig. 6. Z-plasty principle for changing the direction of a linear scar within its central limb by triangular flap transposition.

squares, and/or semicircles in any combination so the scar is harder for the observer's eye to follow.[10] Both geometric closure and W-plasty allow for the contractile forces to fall into the RSTLs in various directions and help camouflage the scar (**Fig. 9**). These scar revision techniques are described in more detail in other articles in this issue corresponding to each facial subunit.

POSTPROCEDURE INCISIONAL CARE
Taping

Randomized controlled trials have shown that applying paper tape to an incision can reduce after incisional scarring.[11] Micropore paper tape is a good choice, which applies pressure to the wound and prevents widening of the incision. Flesh-colored paper tape can blend in with the patients' skin more than white paper tape. Paper tape can be applied for several months, especially in mobile facial regions to prevent widening of the scar.

Moisture

During the healing process to improve re-epithelialization, it is widely accepted that moisture enhances incisional closure.[12] Any moisturizing ointment can be used until full epithelialization has occurred. However, in up to 15% of the population using topical antibiotic ointments longer than 1 week, an increased risk for topical dermatitis exists. Thus, the authors prefer using a more inert petroleum ointment (such as Aquaphor) after the first week.

Silicone Ointments

Once re-epithelialization of the incision is complete, the choice of what topical scar product is used is often subjectively based on physician and patient preference.[13] Topical silicone products have been proven to minimize scarring in randomized, prospective clinical trials. Topical silicone gel or silicone sheeting decreases hypertrophic scar and keloid formation during scar maturation in patients who are at high risk for developing such scars. However, it is unclear that silicone is effective in improving scars in patients who are not at increased risk for significant scarring. The mechanism of action is thought to be that topical silicone increases dermal hydration, thus modulating the growth factor milieu in the skin. In a prospective, randomized control trial of patients undergoing outpatient dermatologic surgery, silicone gel was used twice a day for 2 months after suture removal. The treatment group had a statistical reduction of keloid and hypertrophic scar formation and also reduced symptoms from the healing process (ie, paresthesias, pulling sensations, and alterations in color).[14] Topical vitamin E and onion extract (Mederma) have been shown to minimize scarring in randomized, prospective clinical trials.[15]

Sun Protection

Sun protection plays an important role in reducing a scar's appearance. Topical zinc oxide ointment

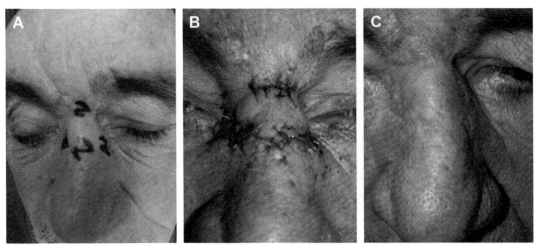

Fig. 7. Z-plasty design with concentric Z-plasties on a patient's nose to smooth out a trap door deformity from a paramedian forehead island ski flap. (*A*) Preoperative photo with planned z-plasty markings. (*B*) Immediate postoperative photo with four z-plasties performed. (*C*) Postoperative photo 6 months later.

has been shown to decrease scar hypertrophy and hyperpigmentation.[16] Sun block greater than 30 sun protection factor is beneficial to reduce pigmentary changes, because it is important to protect vulnerable, new healing tissue from the damaging effects of UV light. The patient should be counseled to avoid sun exposure to the healing site for several months and begin using daily sunscreen 1 month after full epithelialization has occurred even during overcast days.

ADJUNCTIVE PROCEDURES
Dermabrasion

Dermabrasion can improve a scar by making it look more blended with the surrounding tissues. The ideal time to perform dermabrasion is approximately 6 to 8 weeks after the procedure. At this point, the scar is still remodeling and fibroblastic activity is still occurring. Typical dermabrasion is performed at 10,000 to 15,000 rpm down to the papillary-reticular layer of the dermis. Dermabrasion can be useful in improving surface contour irregularities. If a patient is taking oral isotretinoin for acne, dermabrasion or any ablative laser resurfacing procedure should be delayed for at least 1 year due to delayed epithelialization.[17]

Laser

Laser therapy is another adjunctive procedure that is commonly used to improve scar appearance. Laser resurfacing works by increasing collagen remodeling. Laser therapy can be used 6 to 8 weeks after a procedure. Typical lasers used for scar improvement include CO_2, YAG, and pulse dye, which are described in more detail in the other articles in this issue.

The decision of laser versus dermabrasion treatment is based on patient and physician preference. Compared with laser, dermabrasion is lower in cost. However, the result from dermabrasion is more surgeon dependent than the laser. Lasers are more effective in treating hyperpigmentation and should be used with caution in Fitzpatrick III or greater skin types. Dermabrasion is better at improving surface contour irregularities.

POTENTIAL FUTURE SCAR TREATMENTS

In the literature, most scar studies have focused on scar treatment rather than the prevention of postsurgical scars. Future strategies to reduce scars have investigated antiproliferative cytokines (such transforming growth factor β-3, TGF-β-3). Specifically, recombinant human TGF B-3, also known as avotermin (Juvista, Renovo), has shown promise to reduce scarring by intradermal injection compared with controls in several double-blind, placebo controlled clinical trials.[18] This approach is based on the fact that TGF-β-3 inhibits collagen formation and extracellular matrix deposition. When TGF-β-3 was given before and after wounding in full-thickness human skin incisions, in phase I and II clinical trials in Europe, improved scar appearance and less histologic scarring were seen. However, in phase

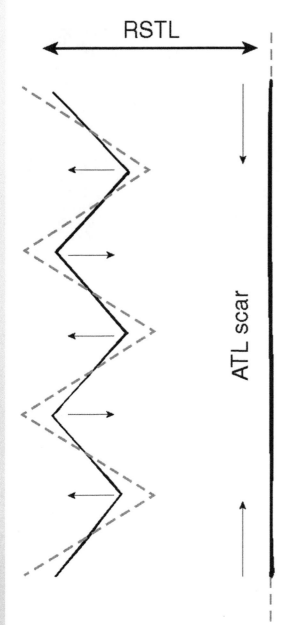

Fig. 8. A W-plasty causes a zigzag pattern modifying the skin contractile forces to be more at right angles to the original linear scar contraction. This allows the scar contractile force to fall within and parallel to the RSTL. ATL, antitension line. (*Adapted from* Borges A. W-plasty in facial scars incision. In: Thomas JR, Holt GR, editors. Revision and camouflage. St Louis (MO): CV Mosby; 1989.)

3, trial therapeutic endpoints were not achieved. Despite this recent result, the concept of prophylactically administering cytokines before and during wounding to reduce scarring remains an intriguing future strategy.[18]

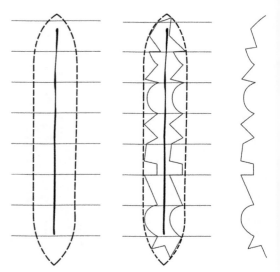

Fig. 9. Design of geometric broken line closure.

SUMMARY

Scarring is an inevitable result after surgery. Scars on the face are clearly visible to the public, and thus, its appearance can be very disconcerting to the patient. By instituting the initial principles of scar management before the procedure, managing patient expectations, and minimizing patient factors that may increase scarring, the best possible scar outcome can be achieved. During the procedure, it is important to use atraumatic tissue handling and proper suture techniques to give the most optimal healing. Designing incisions parallel to RSTLs, or in borders of the facial subunits, makes them less noticeable. Postoperative wound care includes moisturization, taping, sun protection, and possibly topical silicone. Adjunctive procedures such as laser and dermabrasion can be used to improve the final look of the scar during the healing process. The patient should be informed that it requires at least 6 to 12 months for a dermal scar to fully mature. By applying these principles, the degree of facial scarring will be minimized.

REFERENCES

1. Bock O, Schmid-Ott G, Malewski P, et al. Quality of life of patients with keloid and hypertrophic scarring. Arch Dermatol Res 2006;297(10):433–8.
2. PA H. Skin wound healing. In: Hom DB HP, Gosain AK, Friedman DC, editors. Essential tissue healing of the face and neck. Ontario (Canada): B.C. Decker Inc; 2009. p. 1–15.
3. Jefferson GD. Dynamic wound healing. In: Johnson JT, Rosen CA, editors. In: CAR, editor. Bailey's head and neck surgery- otolaryngology, Vol. 1,

5th edition. Baltimore (MD): Lippincott Williams, & Wilkins; 2014. p. 109–19.

4. Leake D. Scar revision and local flap refinement. In: Baker S, editor. Local flaps in facial reconstrucion. Philadelphia: Elselvier; 2007. p. 723–60.

5. Hom DB, Odland R. Prognosis for facial scarring. In: Harahap M, editor. Surgical techniques for cutaneous scar revision. New York: Marcel Decker; 2000. p. 25–37.

6. Visscher MO, Bailey JK, Hom DB. Scar treatment variations by skin type. Facial Plast Surg Clin North Am 2014;22(3):453–62.

7. Lorenz HPLM. Wound healing: repair biology and wound and scar treatment. In: Mathes SJ, editor. Plastic surgery. Philadelphia: Elsevier Inc.; 2006. p. 209–34.

8. Borges A. Pre-operative planning for better incisional scars. In: Regan Thomas J, Holt GR, editors. Facial scar—incision, revision, and camouflage. St Louis (MO): Mosby; 1989. p. 41–56.

9. Perez-Bustillo A, Gonzalez-Sixto B, Rodriguez-Prieto MA. Surgical principles for achieving a functional and cosmetically acceptable scar. Actas dermosifiliogr 2013;104(1):17–28.

10. Rodgers BJ, Williams EF, Hove CR. W-plasty and geometric broken line closure. Facial Plast Surg 2001;17(4):239–44.

11. Atkinson JA, McKenna KT, Barnett AG, et al. A randomized, controlled trial to determine the efficacy of paper tape in preventing hypertrophic scar formation in surgical incisions that traverse Langer's skin tension lines. Plast Reconstr Surg 2005;116(6): 1648–56 [discussion 1657–8].

12. Winter GD. Formation of the scab and the rate of epithelization of superficial wounds in the skin of the young domestic pig. Nature 1962;193:293–4.

13. Hom DB, Hom KA. Do topical products reduce post-incision scars? Laryngoscope 2015;125(2):282–3.

14. de Giorgi V, Sestini S, Mannone F, et al. The use of silicone gel in the treatment of fresh surgical scars: a randomized study. Clin Exp Dermatol 2009;34(6): 688–93.

15. Khoo TL, Halim AS, Zakaria Z, et al. A prospective, randomised, double-blinded trial to study the efficacy of topical tocotrienol in the prevention of hypertrophic scars. J Plast Reconstr Aesthet Surg 2011; 64(6):e137–45.

16. Aksoy B, Atakan N, Aksoy HM, et al. Effectiveness of topical zinc oxide application on hypertrophic scar development in rabbits. Burns 2010;36(7):1027–35.

17. Koranda FC. Dermabrasion in facial scars incision, revision and camouflage. In: Thomas JR, Holt GR, editors. Facial scar—incision, revision, and camouflage. St Louis (MO): CV Mosby; 1989. p. 123–36.

18. So K, McGrouther DA, Bush JA, et al. Avotermin for scar improvement following scar revision surgery: a randomized, double-blind, within-patient, placebo-controlled, phase II clinical trial. Plast Reconstr Surg 2011;128(1):163–72.

Management of Forehead Scars

Ryan Heffelfinger, MD[a],*, Akshay Sanan, MD[b], Lucas M. Bryant, MD[b]

KEYWORDS

- Wound healing • Scars • Forehead • Facial plastic surgery • Laser • Filler • Reconstruction
- Eyebrow

KEY POINTS

- The homogenous topography of the forehead makes the creation of inconspicuous scars challenging.
- Careful preoperative planning, open communication, and setting realistic expectations are vital to any scar revision case.
- Use natural borders (hairline, brow, temporal line, facial rhytids) to disguise scars whenever possible. Hair transplant can help restore appearance when scars involve hair-bearing skin.
- Protection of function always takes priority over restoration of form.
- Convex, contracted scars may benefit from injection of filler, including fat transfer.

INTRODUCTION

Injuries to the forehead pose several challenges to the facial plastic and reconstructive surgeon. Some of these challenges are held in common with other facial regions, and others are unique. This article is designed to take the reader through an organized, stepwise approach to acute and chronic scar management of the forehead region. Forehead wounds may present for a variety of reasons, including facial trauma, defects remaining after excision of malignant or nonmalignant lesions, the result of congenital facial lesions, and from iatrogenic causes.

Reconstruction of forehead wounds can be approached using a standardized and complete methodology. Repair may range from local wound care, primary closure, local tissue rearrangement, regional flap reconstruction and complex free tissue transfer, or any combination thereof. In addition to optimizing the patient's aesthetic appearance, goals of repair include protection of vital structures, prevention of infection, and avoidance of chronic wound complications.

Successful reconstruction depends on several synergistic factors. The nature of the wound, careful preoperative planning, surgical competence, and the global medical status of the patient all play a role. When one of these pillars of wound repair are lacking, the others become even more important. Patients who smoke, have vasculopathy, or are not medically stable to undergo an intensive procedure may have limited options for repair. The importance of this concept cannot be emphasized enough for the neophyte surgeon. Patients may require serial procedures (in the case of tissue expander use, for example), and the possibility of this should be discussed up front. Depending on the nature of their injury, patients may remain significantly disfigured, even after the

Disclosures: None of the authors listed above have anything to disclose.
[a] Division of Facial Plastic & Reconstructive Surgery, Department of Otolaryngology – Head & Neck Surgery, Thomas Jefferson University Hospital, Thomas Jefferson University, 925 Chestnut Street, 7th Floor, Philadelphia, PA 19107, USA; [b] Department of Otolaryngology – Head & Neck Surgery, Thomas Jefferson University Hospital, Thomas Jefferson University, 925 Chestnut Street, 6th Floor, Philadelphia, PA 19107, USA
* Corresponding author.
E-mail address: Ryan.Heffelfinger@jefferson.edu

best possible reconstructive effort has been executed well. It is vital for the surgeon to maintain open and honest communication with the patient throughout the reconstructive journey.

A scar is the final, unavoidable result of any wound, whether it is repaired masterfully or neglected in its entirety. Facial scarring can be particularly troublesome to patients because it is something the patient and those they encounter will see on a daily basis. Even if vital structures have been protected and function restored, an unappealing facial scar can cause persistent and significant emotional suffering in patients.[1] Surgeons can minimize the impact of facial scarring on a patient through careful planning and the use of optimal reconstructive measures.

Scars are fluid, evolving over time. They change in color when healing and when exposed to various environmental factors such as sunlight or a chemical irritant. They change in shape when exposed to tension or movement during wound healing. Although the strength of a scar builds over time, it will never regain the full resilience of native tissue. Last, scars are subject to hereditary forces. Some patient's wound healing may be burdened with the challenges of dyschromias, scar hypertrophy, or keloid reactions over time. The successful facial plastic surgeon uses a broad armamentarium to address the unique needs of each patient and optimize final outcomes.

MANAGEMENT AND TREATMENT
Overview

Scar management begins at the time of cutaneous insult. Wounds should be cleaned, and copious irrigation used. Anesthesia (local, intravenous, or general) may be needed for adequate debridement and examination. Never allow treatable patient discomfort to limit one's initial examination.[2] Depending on the wound class, antibiotics may be indicated. In cases of polytrauma, where the facial wound is not a singular injury, cooperation with several other treatment teams may be necessary. When forehead wounds are the result of a surgical excision, these primary steps may have already occurred.

In comparison with other facial regions, the forehead is relatively devoid of geometric complexity. Any aberration of the symmetric, gentle contour, and homogenous appearance of the forehead readily stands out to the observer. A concave scar within the convex topography of the midforehead can cast shadows and distort light reflection patterns, making an otherwise innocuous scar readily stand out.

A complete understanding of facial anatomy as well as the biomechanical interactions that occur both acutely and over time within the face is a foundational principle in successful facial reconstruction. One of the first things a surgeon should become facile with is facial analysis. Facial analysis helps to define both aesthetic ideals, as well as aberrations. Facial analysis can be performed from many observer views (frontal, oblique, profile), but forehead analysis is often most helpful using the frontal view. One should be careful not to perseverate with exacting geometric definitions at the expense of patient preference and the pursuit of global facial harmony.

All forehead intervention must take into consideration the effects it will have on adjacent key anatomic structures. Forehead tissues are generally unforgiving, and distortion of adjacent subsites is a frequent challenge. It is also important to anticipate future changes, such as the effect of balding on hairline shape and location. A carefully placed scar line within a young male's hairline may become painfully obvious several years later.

Facial Analysis

The facial frame can be divided into subunits both vertically and horizontally. Facial height can be divided into thirds, with the forehead comprising the superior third. The superior third (forehead) is defined as running from trichion to glabella (**Fig. 1**). Although typically described as the superior third, variability in a patient's hairline may result in the forehead subunit comprising significantly more or less than one-third of the overall vertical facial dimension.

The face can also be subdivided into vertical segments using the facial vertical fifths model. This results in 3 unique vertical subunits: midforehead, paramedian, and lateral (temporal; see

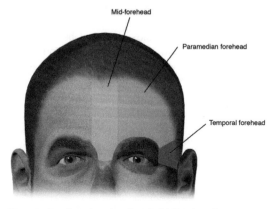

Fig. 1. Forehead subunits (mid-forehead, paramedian, temple).

Fig. 1). The lateral forehead subunit is concave in shape. It is bordered by the hairline posterosuperiorly and the temporal line and lateral orbital rim anteriorly. The paramedian forehead region is bordered superiorly by the hairline, and inferiorly by the superior orbital rim and overlying brow. The mid-forehead region is bound superiorly by the hairline (including the trichion), and inferiorly by the glabella and nasal root (nasion, sellion, and rhinion).

Mid-Forehead

When using the facial fifths model of facial analysis, the mid-fifth describes the mid-forehead region. It is the only nonpaired subunit of the forehead. Its topography is homogenous and it is the most projected subunit of the forehead. The surface anatomy is largely convex in nature. It contains the medial border of both frontalis muscles. The frontalis is the anterior muscle belly of the occipitofrontalis muscle. Owing to the lack of frontalis muscle in the midline, the mid-forehead region is amenable to either vertical or midline scars. This region contains both horizontal rhytids (frontalis, procerus) and vertical rhytids (corrugator supercilii).

Superior mid-forehead defects may be closed with advancement flaps. Trichophytic incisions, or those placed within the hairline (as would be done for a coronal approach), may be used to gain further tissue laxity. An example of this is an O-T rotational flap to close a superior mid-forehead defect adjacent to the hairline. Midline vertically oriented scars may be less likely to undergo scar widening owing to the lack of frontalis muscle activity during healing. Inverted V–Y advancement flaps may help to obviate eyebrow medialization with primary closure of glabellar wounds.[3]

Paramedian Forehead

The paramedian forehead is bordered inferiorly by the superior orbital rim, laterally by the temporal line, and medially by the border of brow/canthus. Notable skeletal landmarks include the prominence of the supraorbital rim. The majority of sensory innervation of the forehead is provided via terminal branches of the ophthalmic division (V_1) of the trigeminal nerve. The supratrochlear neurovascular bundle lies medial to the supraorbital neurovascular bundle and runs beneath the corrugator supercilii and frontalis muscles. The supraorbital notch, which may be palpated along the superior orbital rim, lies approximately at the junction of the mid and medial thirds of brow. These nerves are paired with the supraorbital and supratrochlear vessels. In most patients, the supraorbital structures exit via a notch. However, in approximately 10% of the population, the neurovascular structures may exit slightly more superiorly via a true foramen. These patients are at increased risk for injury during dissection. Overlying this is the eyebrow. Although eyebrow hairs do not undergo balding patterns intrinsic to scalp hair, the surgeon should consult the patient regarding facial grooming patterns (shaving, plucking, waxing), because this may alter the brow shape and brow line. This area holds several key neurovascular structures, namely the supratrochlear artery and nerve, and the supraorbital artery and nerves. The inferior border of the paramedian region involves periorbital structures including the brow and upper eyelid.

The degree of bossing of an individual's forehead varies, but the region from the midline to the midpupillary line is convex. The relaxed skin tension lines (RSTLs) in the forehead are horizontal. When possible, horizontally oriented incisions are preferred to allow maximal scar camouflage. Eyebrow elevation is of particular importance in this forehead region. When large defects (>3 cm) are closed primarily in a horizontally oriented plane, the result often yields excessive eyebrow elevation. Defects near the hairline in the paramedian forehead that are closed in a horizontal fashion impact the eyebrow much less compared with inferiorly based defects. When defects will effect eyebrow elevation, the surgeon can limit this by suturing the eyebrow dermis and the underlying muscle to the periosteum of the superior orbital rim.

To minimize scar for defects of the paramedian forehead near the hairline, a bipedicle advancement flap is used. Bipedicle flaps are recruited from tissue superior to the defect and the incision is carried full thickness to the galea. The bipedicled flap is well-vascularized by the subdermal plexus and provides a hidden scar. One of its drawbacks is lowering of the anterior hairline. Of note, the longer the releasing incision for the bipedicled flap, the greater mobility the flap has. Advancement flaps are used to close skin defects in the paramedian forehead, which are not amenable to primary closure. Incisions are made along the horizontal RSTLs. Flaps are made at a 4:1 ratio of length to width and are dissected in the subcutaneous tissue plane, superficial to the neurovascular bundle. Effective dissection in the correct plane, squaring of the defect borders, and removing standing cutaneous deformities is imperative to appropriate scar formation. An effective method to camouflage scar formation is to make the flap slightly wider than necessary to hide incisions in nearby skin creases.

Management of a scar in the paramedian forehead region can be challenging. Thus, attempts should be made by the surgeon to avoid vertical, curvilinear, and oblique incisions because they result in scars that are not in the RSTLs. The majority of defects should be repaired primarily in a horizontal orientation or reconstructed with horizontally oriented unilateral or bilateral advancement flaps. Further, vertically oriented primary repair should be avoided. Rotation and transposition flaps should also be avoided.

In paramedian forehead wounds, which include the brow, additional procedures such as lateral cantholysis may be required to address the integrity of the eyelid.[4] Other options in the brow region include a pedicled forehead flap.[4,5] If a significant amount of tissue loss occurs in the supraorbital region, reconstruction may result in a similar effect as a direct brow lift. In such cases, it is reasonable to consider addressing the contralateral face to maintain symmetry. Periorbital defects extending below the eyebrow are discussed in a different chapter of this text.

A good method for closure of moderate sized defects within the paramedian and temporal region is the hatchet or double hatchet flap (**Fig. 2**). Gurunluoglu and colleagues[5] describe its use within the region for primary closure of defects up to 3.5 cm in maximum diameter while maintaining neurovascular integrity of the region. This flap design allows for optimal rotation and wound coverage, while minimizing tension and distortion of adjacent subunits. The incisions should be designed in such a manner as to align with the hairline and facial rhytids if possible.

Temple Region

The temporal region of the forehead is separated from the lateral border of the paramedian region by the temporal line. The temporal line is an arc of bone, which serves as an attachment point for the temporal fascia. More posteriorly, the temporal line divides into a superior and inferior temporal line, the superior corresponding with temporal fascia insertion and the inferior corresponding with

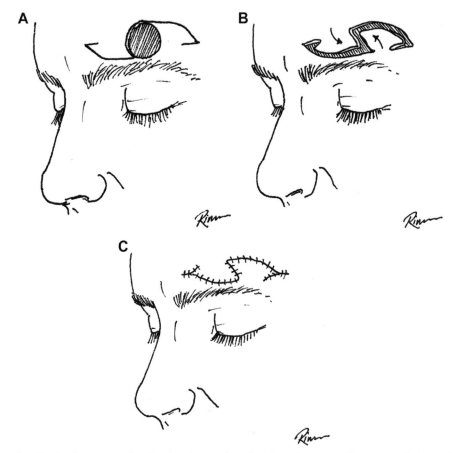

Fig. 2. Hatchet flap in the paramedian forehead. Note how incision placement allows wound closure in the line of the relaxed skin tension lines. (*A*) Schematic rendering of defect and flap. (*B*) Rotating tissue allowing for closure of defect. (*C*) Defect closed. (*Courtesy of* Ryan Rimmer, MD, Philadelphia, PA.)

the origin of the temporalis muscle. The temporal line extends from the parietal bone posteriorly to the posterior border of the zygoma at the frontozygomatic suture line. The mid-forehead and paramedian regions lie anteromedial to the temporal line and are convex in shape.

The temporal region of the forehead lies posterolateral to the temporal line and is predominantly concave. This concavity affords the reconstructive surgeon different reconstructive options when compared with how one may address the convex regions of the forehead. Additionally, there is a relative increase in subcutaneous tissues owing to the volume provided by the temporalis muscle and temporal fat pad.

The temporal region of the forehead is home to several soft tissue structures, including the temporalis muscle. The primary neurovascular structures within the temporal region that are of interest to the reconstructive include the superficial and deep temporal vessels, the frontal branch of the facial nerve, and the sentinel vein. The sentinel vein is a large, zygomaticotemporal perforating vessel between the deep temporal fascia and the temporoparietal fascial layers. It lies approximately 1 cm lateral to the frontozygomatic suture line and sits adjacent to the frontal branch of the facial nerve.[6]

The frontal branch of the facial nerve runs through the temporal region and is responsible for nearly all dynamic movement of the forehead region. It innervates both the periorbital musculature and the frontal division of the occipitofrontalis muscle. The superficial location of the frontal branch of the facial nerve within the temporal region makes it particularly susceptible to injury, even in cases of relatively shallow soft tissue manipulation (**Fig. 3**).

The frontal branch is most at risk for injury as it crosses over the zygoma. The frontal nerve travels in an oblique path. At that level, it lies within the undersurface of the temporoparietal fascia. Several imaginary lines have been described to predict its path across the zygoma. In general, it travels along an imaginary line traveling from the earlobe to 1.5 cm above the lateral border of the eyebrow (Pitanguay's line).[7,8]

Another method of using topographic localization of the frontal branch is described by Sabini and colleagues.[6] They first drew a line from the tragus to the lateral canthus. A second line was then drawn from the bottom of the ear lobe in an oblique fashion, bisecting the first line. This second line was similar in orientation to Pitanguay's line. It was found to associate closely with the course of the facial nerve, but also eliminate the anatomic variability found in patient's eyebrow

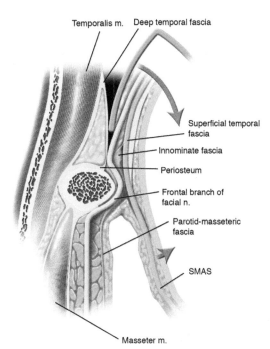

Fig. 3. Frontal branch of the facial nerve relative to the fascial layers of the temporal forehead area. n., nerve; SMAS, superficial musculoaponeurotic system.

position. As the nerve courses medially, it inserts on the deep aspect of the frontalis muscle.

The superficial temporal fascia layer continues as the superficial musculoaponeurotic system inferiorly, and the galea aponeurosis superiorly. This fascial layer contains key neurovascular structures, including the superficial temporal artery, the auriculotemporal nerve, and the frontal branch of the facial nerve.

Reconstructive options within the temporal region include rotational flaps and advancement flaps. Many options used successfully in other forehead regions can be applied in the temporal region as well. Benefits of this region include its relatively increased laxity and concavity. Owing to the concave nature of the temporal region, it is more amenable to skin grafting when other options are insufficient. Skin grafting can also be considered in patients unlikely to tolerate more invasive reconstructive measures.

Scar Management Specific to the Forehead

The first step to a satisfactory outcome with scar revision is a detailed analysis and correct diagnosis of the problem. Scar revision and management involves much more than simply excising a scar and doing a better closure of the wound. Successful scar revision encompasses disguising the fact that a scar is present and tricking the observer's eye into overlooking or ignoring the scar's presence. Additionally, a wide array of techniques must exist within the surgeon's armamentarium, both surgical and nonsurgical, to appropriately manage the high variability of scar presentations. The surgeon's goal should be to select the best technique for the individual patient and scar. The "best technique" tends to be subjective given the relative lack of high-level evidence. It is difficult to produce a well-designed, comparison-controlled trials of various interventions because of differences in objective characterization of scars (color, elevation, texture), and lack of appropriate controls.

Scars can be divided into hypertrophic scars/keloids and nonhypertrophic scars.[9] Hypertrophic scars and keloids are similar in nature and represent an abnormality in wound healing. Histologic findings of hypertrophic scars and keloids include extracellular matrix overproduction and deposition of highly disorganized collagen by fibroblasts. Keloids, by definition, are elevated fibrous scars that extend beyond the borders of the wound and do not regress. Hypertrophic scars tend to develop earlier than keloids (8 vs 12 weeks), are confined to the wound borders, and regress at 12 to 24 months. Nonhypertrophic scars are divided into atrophic (depressed) scars or scars that are flat.

Factors impacting the development of unnecessary scar development include the direction of the scar with respect to RSTLs, distortion of facial subunits, irregular texture to the scar surface, and a color mismatch between the scar and surrounding tissues. Aesthetic borders between or at the margins of facial subunits are excellent locations for incision placement or scar relocation. With respect to the forehead region, these borders include the hairline and eyebrow line. Acknowledgment of RSTLs is important because an incision or closure that crosses these at an angle of greater than 30 to 40° will produce an aesthetically displeasing result. One of the ideal scar camouflage techniques is achieved by placement of incisions within existing skin folds produced by RSTLs.[10,11]

Surgical techniques
Hair transplantation Scars within the forehead region may include hair-bearing skin. Hair transplantation may be considered in such cases to aid in scar camouflage. Because hair transplantation techniques have evolved from large, multifollicular unit "plugs" to follicular units and single follicle micrografts, successful hair transplantation can be nearly indistinguishable from native hair by the casual observer.

The eyebrow can be restored with hair transplantation. Care is made to align the vector of the transplanted follicle with the natural vector of eyebrow hair. Depending on the donor site, the patient should be counseled on the likely need to trim and maintain the transplanted hairs, because they will continue to grow and function in a manner that depends on their site of origin. The process can be time consuming, but good results have been reported.[12]

Z-plasty The Z-plasty transposition flap can provide excellent cosmesis and is used primarily to lengthen the scar, release scar contracture, disrupt a scar, or realign a scar within an RSTL.[13,14] Z-plasty does have its drawbacks, including that lengthening a scar in 1 direction results in shortening in the perpendicular direction. Also, a total of 3 scars are made in place of one. The ultimate effect of a Z-plasty is disruption of the scar itself and reorientation of the scar along the limbs of incisions.

W-plasty The W-plasty is helpful in managing long, straight scars. These scars reflect light homogeneously and are easy for the eye to follow. The W-plasty creates a regularly irregular incision, which allows for light scattering, making the scar less visible to the observer (**Figs. 4** and **5**). Unlike a Z-plasty, this technique does not increase the length of the scar.

Geometric broken line closure Geometric broken line closure (GBLC) produces an irregularly, irregular incision and is more complicated and time consuming than a W-plasty (**Figs. 6** and **7**). This technique is ideally used for scars that are long and angled 45° or greater from RSTLs. GBLC incorporates a series of advancement flaps in the form of opposing semicircles, squares,

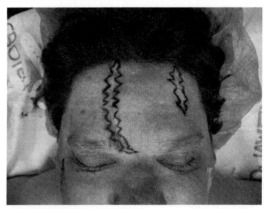

Fig. 4. Preoperative marking of W-plasty in 2 long, vertical paramedian forehead scars.

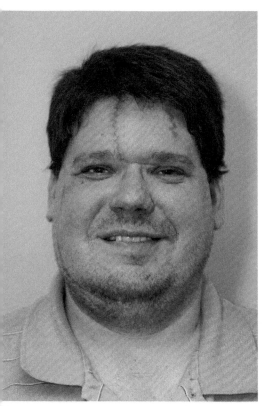

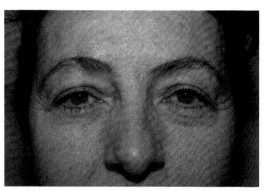

Fig. 7. Postoperative picture of a patient after a geometric broken line closure of a paramedian forehead scar.

Fig. 5. 2 week postoperative picture of a patient after a W-plasty of 2 paramedian forehead scars. The redness of the scar is normal postoperative wound healing.

rhomboids, triangles, and rectangles in varying order and size. The key feature of this technique is the randomness of its design, which is difficult for the observer to track. Thus, GBLC is useful for lengthy and irregular scars of the forehead. The GBLC design is excised under tension taking the interposing skin and scar.

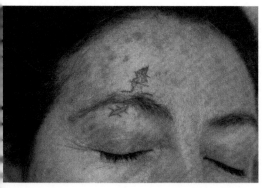

Fig. 6. Preoperative marking of geometric broken line closure of a paramedian forehead scar. Note the scar traverses the eyebrow.

Nonsurgical and adjunctive techniques Although surgery is the mainstay of treatment for scars in the forehead region, nonsurgical and adjunct modalities should be part of the surgeon's armamentarium. These techniques can be used as monotherapies in the appropriate clinical setting. This section reviews the various nonsurgical and adjunctive techniques to forehead scars.

Steroids Steroids continue to be a good option for scar management, camouflage, and revision in the forehead region. The mechanism of action is believed to be the suppression and reduction of collagen cross-linking and deposition, thus preventing further scar formation. Steroids injected intralesionally have been shown to decrease the elevation and erythema of scars, which can be used immediately after surgical closure and also as a primary intervention. Steroids are used as first-line treatment for both hypertrophic scars and keloids. The most commonly used steroid is triamcinolone acetonide (Kenalog, Delcor Asset Corporation, Lake Forest, IL). Triamcinolone injections have been shown to flatten small keloids by 50% to 100% and decrease their rate of recurrence.[15] The recurrence rates improve more when intralesional steroid injection is coupled with other modalities including silicone sheeting and/or surgical excision. Earlier steroid injections also yield superior outcomes with regard to scar prevention. The side effects of steroid injection include hypopigmentation, pain at site of injection, dermal and adipose atrophy, and, rarely, tissue necrosis.[16]

Laser resurfacing Lasers have been widely used for scar management.[9] Lasers can be used as monotherapy or as an adjunct to surgery and other nonsurgical techniques. Lasers are divided into ablative and nonablative, depending on depth of penetration and based on wavelength and absorption. Both types of lasers play a role in scar management and their use can be used in management of forehead scars. All lasers should be used judiciously in patients with skin types Fitzpatrick IV to VI because of an increased side effect profile, primarily irreversible hypopigmentation.

The 2 most commonly used ablative lasers are the CO_2 laser and the Er:YAG laser. The absorbing chromophore for both lasers is water. Both lasers increase thermal energy, which results in vaporization. Ablative lasers are known to yield good results for treating hypertrophic scars and keloids (**Figs. 8** and **9**). Ablative lasers can be used as monotherapy, but superior results are appreciated when combined with intralesional steroid injection. Er:YAG causes less tissue necrosis than CO_2 and may be better suited for scar margins. Disadvantages to ablative lasers include pain, prolonged down time, persistent erythema up to 3 months, increased risk for viral and bacterial infections, hyperpigmentation, and hypopigmentation. Er:YAG has a lesser likelihood of these problems compared with CO_2 because it can be applied more precisely and has a greater affinity for water. Fractionated CO_2 lasers also have a

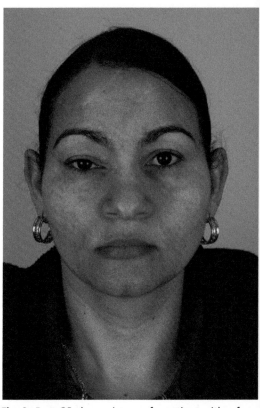

Fig. 9. Post-CO_2 laser picture of a patient with a forehead scar. Note the flattening and depigmentation of the scar.

better safety profile and lesser downtime when compared with traditional CO_2 lasers.[17] It should be noted that some of the benefits of these lasers, namely, the elimination of dyschromias, may cause abnormal pigmentation patterns and the treatment of the entire forehead, or even the entire face, may provide the optimal aesthetic results.

Nonablative lasers include the 585-nm pulsed dye laser and Nd:YAG laser. The main chromophore is oxyhemoglobin in the microvasculature, which leads to targeted vaporization and subsequent tissue ischemia. Intracellular water is not affected (compared with ablative lasers), thus no tissue necrosis is noted. The net result is a leveling of the scar with decreased erythema. Nonablative lasers have also been shown to stimulate extracellular matrix deposition, which makes these lasers desirable for depressed or atrophic scars. Nonablative lasers are also used to treat hyperpigmented scars. Disadvantages to nonablative lasers include downtime, erythema, and an increased risk for viral and bacterial infections.[18]

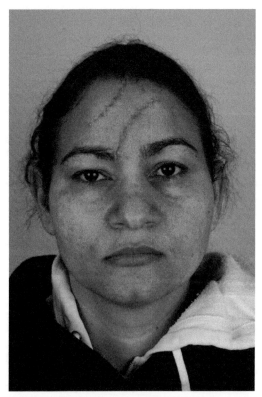

Fig. 8. Pre-CO_2 laser picture of a patient with a raised, erythematous forehead scar.

Dermabrasion Dermabrasion can be used as a nonsurgical treatment for forehead scars. The goal of dermabrasion is to level the skin of a hypertrophic scar or keloid while also promoting reepithelialization and extracellular matrix deposition. Dermabrasion classically has been used for acne scarring and rhinophyma, but can be used after surgery to smooth uneven scars. Care must be taken to injure the epithelium to the level of the papillary dermis as the reticular dermis maintains the structures, which will promote reepithelialization.

Intralesional fillers Injectable fillers are very useful for atrophic scars in the forehead region. They function as a means of direct scar camouflage. Fillers can be autologous (fat), allogenic, xenogenic, or synthetic. Of note, fillers may elicit a foreign body or inflammatory response after injection, which may paradoxically cause hypertrophic changes. Thus, patients must be counseled on the potential for superficial skin changes or granuloma formation. Neurovascular anatomy and patterns in the forehead must be appreciated, because necrosis owing to intravascular injection has been described in the forehead region.

Botulinum toxin An increasing body of evidence suggests that botulinum toxin–induced immobilization of forehead wounds results in enhanced wound healing.[19,20] The forehead is a particularly favorable area to treat because of its low associated risk of inducing temporary functional deficits. Botulinum toxin temporarily weakens surrounding muscles, thus lessening the pull on the wound during the acute healing phase of the first 2 to 4 months. By paralyzing nearby muscles, botulinum toxin helps to prevent the development of a wide scar (**Figs. 10** and **11**). As a general principle, the senior author advises all patients undergoing scar revision in the forehead region receive botulinum toxin injection 2 weeks before surgery.

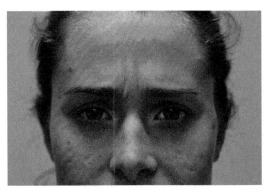

Fig. 11. Mid-forehead scar worsens with muscle contraction. This patient is a good candidate for Botox injection.

ACKNOWLEDGMENTS

The authors thank Ryan Rimmer, MD, Resident Physician, Thomas Jefferson University, Department of Otolaryngology – Head & Neck Surgery for the illustration of double hatchet flap (see **Fig. 2**).

REFERENCES

1. Levine Elie, Degutis L, Pruzinsky T, et al. Quality of life and facial trauma: psychological and body image effects. Ann Plast Surg 2005;54(5):502–10.
2. Bryant L, Heffelfinger R, Pribitkin E. Management of acute facial soft tissue injuries. In: Sclafani A, editor. Sataloff's comprehensive textbook of otolaryngology: head & neck surgery (facial plastic and reconstructive surgery) - volume 3, vol. 3, 1st edition. Philadelphia: Jaypee; 2016. p. 1. Print.
3. Baker S. Local flaps in facial reconstruction. Third edition, Vol. 3. Elsevier; 2014.
4. Ozkaya Mutlu O, Egemen O, Dilber A, et al. Aesthetic unit-based reconstruction of periorbital defects. J Craniofac Surg 2016;27(2):429–32. Web.
5. Gurunluoglu R, Shafighi M, Williams SA, et al. Reconstruction of large supra-eyebrow and forehead defects using the hatchet flap principle and sparing sensory nerve branches. Ann Plast Surg 2012;68(1):37–42. Web.
6. Sabini P, Wayne I, Quatela VC. Anatomical guides to precisely localize the frontal branch of the facial nerve. Arch Facial Plast Surg 2003;5(2):150–2. Web.
7. Pitanguy I, Ramos AS. The frontal branch of the facial nerve: the importance of its variations in face lifting. Plast Reconstr Surg 1966;38:352–6.
8. Raposio E, PierLuigi S, Nordstrom RE. Effects of galeotomies on scalp flaps. Ann Plast Surg 1998;41(1): 17–21.
9. Lee Y. Combination treatment of surgical, post-traumatic and post-herpetic scars with ablative lasers

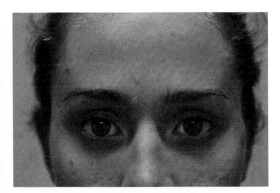

Fig. 10. Patient with scar in right glabella.

followed by fractional laser and non-ablative laser in Asians. Lasers Surg Med 2009;41(2):131–40.

10. Clark JM, Wang TD. Local flaps in scar revision. Facial Plast Surg 2001;17(4):295–308.

11. Schweinfurth JM, Fedok F. Avoiding pitfalls and unfavorable outcomes in scar revision. Facial Plast Surg 2001;17(4):273–8.

12. Goldman GD. Eyebrow transplantation. Dermatol Surg 2001;27(4):352–4.

13. Hove CR, Williams EF III, Rodgers BJ. Z-plasty: a concise review. Facial Plast Surg 2001;17(4):289–94.

14. Igde M, Yilanci S, Bali YY, et al. Reconstruction of tissue defects developing after excision of non-melanoma malignant skin tumors in scalp and forehead regions. Turk Neurosurg 2015;25(6)):888–94. Web.

15. Juckett G, Hartman-Adams H. Management of keloids and hypertrophic scars. Am Fam Physician 2009;80(3):253–60.

16. Capon A, Iarmarcovai G, Gonnelli D, et al. Scar prevention using laser-assisted skin healing (LASH) in plastic surgery. Aesthetic Plast Surg 2010;34(4):438–46.

17. Elsaie ML, Choudhary S. Lasers for scars: a review and evidence-based appraisal. J Drugs Dermatol 2010;9(11):1355–62.

18. Alster TS, Tanzi EL, Lazarus M. The use of fractional laser photothermolysis for the treatment of atrophic scars. Dermatol Surg 2007;33(3):295–9.

19. Sherris DA, Gassner HG. Botulinum toxin to minimize facial scarring. Facial Plast Surg 2002;18(1):35–9.

20. Siegle R. Reconstruction of the Forehead. In: Baker S, editor. Local flaps in facial reconstruction. 3rd edition. Philadelphia: Elsevier Saunders; 2014. p. 563–88. Print.

Periorbital Scar Correction

Christopher B. Chambers, MD[a], Kristen S. Moe, MD[b,c],*

KEYWORDS

- Eyelid retraction • Entropion • Ectropion • Periorbital scar • Eyelid cicatrix

KEY POINTS

- Eyelid reconstruction must respect the anterior and posterior lamella.
- Proper identification of the anatomic cause of cicatrix guides treatment.
- Appropriate graft selection for eyelid retraction repair is paramount to maintaining proper eyelid function and protection of the eye.
- 5-Fluorouacil mixed with Kenalog injected into the retracted eyelid can be an effective treatment modality for periorbital scarring.

INTRODUCTION

Scar formation around the eyes can be aesthetically unpleasing but can also have serious consequences if not appropriately treated. Correction of eyelid and adnexal tissue presents a unique challenge: not only must defects be corrected but the delicate balance of the support system maintaining the position of the eyelids must be restored and augmented against the contractile forces that occur during healing. Even minor disturbances in the three-dimensional forces that act on the eyelids can lead to debilitating malposition and highly visible esthetic deformity.

As a result, scarring of the eyelid can cause eyelid retraction, entropion, and ectropion, which in turn can lead to exposure keratopathy, corneal scarring, infection, blindness, and even perforation of the globe. Periocular scarring can be one of the most challenging conditions facing surgeons who operate in this area, and a thorough understanding of eyelid anatomy as well as function are essential for proper reconstruction of the lid.

ANATOMY

The function of the eyelids is to lubricate and protect the cornea and conjunctival surface. Incomplete closure or lagophthalmos can lead to ocular surface decompensation and vision loss. The lower eyelid should rest at the inferior limbus and the upper eyelid should sit 1 to 2 mm below the superior limbus with the eye open.[1] Scleral show, or visualization of the sclera above or below the limbus, suggests upper or lower eyelid retraction respectively.

One of the most important anatomic concepts for eyelid surgery is the anterior and posterior lamella, which can be separated along the gray line on the lid margin. Some investigators describe a middle lamella, making the eyelid a trilaminar structure. Reconstruction without respect and attention to these structures is likely to result in unfavorable outcomes. The anterior lamella is composed of the skin and orbicularis muscle (**Fig. 1**). The skin of the eyelid has no subcutaneous fat and is the thinnest skin in the body. The

[a] Division of Oculoplastic Surgery, Department of Ophthalmology, University of Washington School of Medicine, Seattle, WA, USA; [b] Division of Facial Plastic and Reconstructive Surgery, Department of Otolaryngology, University of Washington School of Medicine, Seattle, WA, USA; [c] Division of Facial Plastic and Reconstructive Surgery, Department of Neurological Surgery, University of Washington School of Medicine, Seattle, WA, USA
* Corresponding author. Division of Facial Plastic and Reconstructive Surgery, Department of Otolaryngology, University of Washington School of Medicine, Seattle, WA.
E-mail address: krismoe@u.washington.edu

Facial Plast Surg Clin N Am 25 (2017) 25–36
http://dx.doi.org/10.1016/j.fsc.2016.08.007
1064-7406/17/© 2016 Elsevier Inc. All rights reserved.

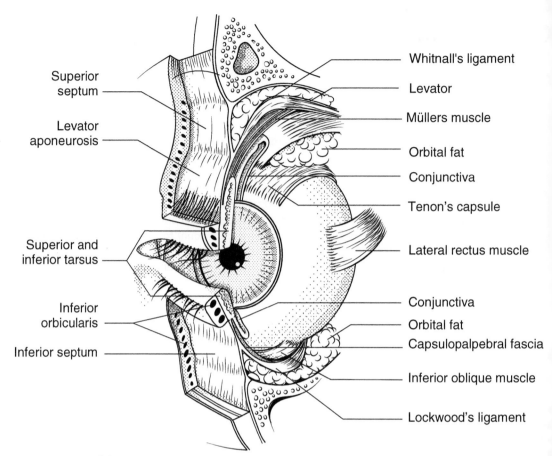

Superior septum

Levator aponeurosis

Superior and inferior tarsus

Inferior orbicularis

Inferior septum

Whitnall's ligament

Levator

Müllers muscle

Orbital fat

Conjunctiva

Tenon's capsule

Lateral rectus muscle

Conjunctiva

Orbital fat

Capsulopalpebral fascia

Inferior oblique muscle

Lockwood's ligament

Fig. 1. Anatomy of the upper and lower eyelids.

orbicularis oculi muscle is the protractor of the eyelid and is divided into the pretarsal, preseptal, and orbital portions. The pretarsal and preseptal portions are responsible for involuntary closure of the lid, whereas the orbital portion is responsible for forced closure. Scarring of the anterior lamella often leads to eyelid retraction and/or eyelid ectropion.

The posterior lamella consists of the tarsus and conjunctiva. The conjunctiva is a nonkeratinized mucous membrane that lines the eyelid and the sclera. It contains goblet cells that secrete mucus to lubricate the eye as well as accessory lacrimal glands that contribute to the aqueous layer of the tear film. There is redundancy of the conjunctiva deep in the fornix to allow proper movement of the globe. Scarring of the conjunctiva and symblepharon formation can cause restriction of the eye, resulting in diplopia. The tarsus is located anterior to and firmly adherent to the conjunctiva. The tarsal plates are formed of dense fibrous connective tissue and provide structural integrity to the lids. The height of the tarsus in the upper eyelid is around 8 to 12 mm and 3.5 to 5 mm in the lower lid.[2] The tarsus tapers

medially and laterally before condensing in to the medial and lateral canthal tendon respectively. Scarring of the posterior lamella can lead to eyelid retraction and/or entropion.

The middle lamella consists of the tissue between the anterior and posterior lamella inferior to the tarsal plate, which includes the orbital septum, the preaponeurotic fat pad, and the lower eyelid retractors. Scarring of the middle lamella can cause eyelid retraction, entropion, and even ectropion. Scarring of the middle lamella is often caused by trauma or surgery.

The medial and lateral canthal tendons attach the tarsal plate to the periosteum of the orbital rim, providing support for the eyelid (**Fig. 2**). The medial canthal tendon separates into an anterior and posterior portion. The anterior portion extends to the anterior lacrimal crest on the frontal bone and provides the major support for the medial canthal angle.[3,4] The posterior portion inserts on the posterior lacrimal crest and provides posterior tension on the eyelid, maintaining close approximation to the globe.[5] The anterior and posterior portions of the medial canthal tendon surround

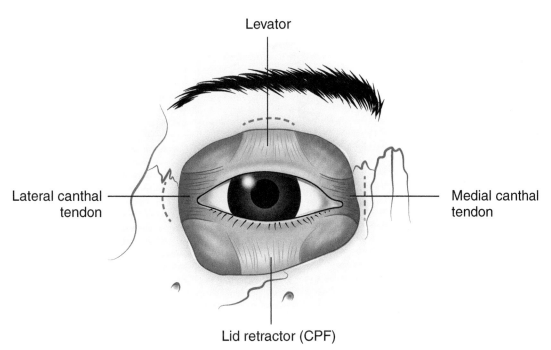

Levator

Lateral canthal
tendon

Medial canthal
tendon

Lid retractor (CPF)

Fig. 2. The support system of the upper and lower eyelids consisting of the medial and lateral canthal tendons, the levator aponeurosis and the capsulopalpebral fascia (CPF).

the lacrimal sac and play an important role in the lacrimal pump mechanism. Any reconstruction of the medial canthal tendon should respect the lacrimal drainage system and be designed to provide appropriate support and posterior tension.

The lateral canthal tendon provides support of the lateral eyelid and inserts at the lateral orbital (Whitnall) tubercle 3 to 4 mm deep to the lateral palpebral raphe.[6] The posterior insertion of the lateral canthal tendon is important to recreate during reconstruction to provide adequate contact between the eyelid and globe. The lateral canthus lies 2 to 4 mm higher than the medial canthus (with some variation by age and race) and periorbital scarring can distort this cosmetically and functionally important upward slant to the eyelid.[7]

EVALUATION

The goal of scar revision and eyelid reconstruction is to provide a functional and aesthetically pleasing result. Often these two outcome goals are related. Evaluation of the scarring and retraction should identify the cause of retraction. The lid should be evaluated for anterior lamellar shortening, posterior lamellar shortening, middle lamellar shortening, canthal tendon laxity, or a combination of these variables. Eyelid retraction may present as an entropion, ectropion, or simply as eyelid retraction. Identification of the anatomic abnormality is paramount to proper scar revision and retraction repair.

The 2-finger test (**Fig. 3**C) is useful to help identify the disorder causing the eyelid retraction. In this test, 2 fingers are placed on the skin below the eyelid and the skin is elevated superiorly. This test provides extra anterior lamellar skin to the periorbital area. When applying superior traction to the skin, pay attention to the eyelid margin. If after elevation of the skin, the lid moves superiorly and the retraction is resolved, the cause of retraction is likely deficiency of the anterior lamella. If the lid does not move and the traction remains despite providing adequate skin to the lid, the retraction is likely caused by posterior or middle lamellar cicatrix.

The laxity of the eyelid must also be considered when evaluating eyelid retraction. The cause of eyelid malposition may be canthal tendon weakness. In many cases there is a combination of lid laxity as well as lamellar shortening and both pathologic states must be addressed for proper repair. The lower lid distraction (**Fig. 3**B, I) can be used to measure lid laxity. In this test, the lid is pulled anteriorly away from the globe and a distraction of greater than 6 mm is considered abnormal. The snap back test can also be used to test for lower lid laxity. The lid is pupped away from the globe and released. The lid should return to its position on the globe without blinking.

Another helpful examination technique for evaluating eyelid malposition is using a finger to place lateral traction on the lid. If lateral tension on the

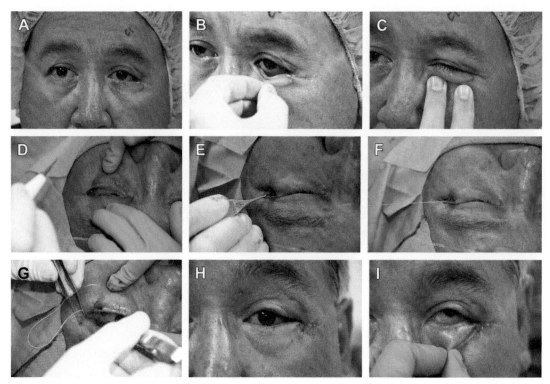

Fig. 3. (*A*) Preoperative appearance, (*B*) snap test, and (*C*) 2-finger test. (*D*) Canthotomy and inferior cantholysis, (*E*) dissection and trimming of lateral tarsal strip, (*F*) suture placed through lateral tarsus for fixation to the periorbital within the medial aspect of the lateral orbit in the region of the Whitnall tubercle (*G*). (*H*) Appearance immediately postoperatively with resolution of lid malposition, and (*I*) normalization of snap test.

lid corrects an observed entropion or ectropion the eyelid malposition may be caused by eyelid laxity and possibly disinsertion of the eyelid retractors.

Ectropion occurs when the eyelid margin everts from the globe. This condition can be caused by cicatricial change, paralysis of the orbicularis muscle, or can be involutional, and can result in excessive evaporation of the tear film and epiphora. Applying the examination techniques discussed earlier can be helpful to identify the cause and direct treatment. If the 2-finger test is applied and the lid margin remains retracted, the ectropion is likely caused by a middle lamellar deficiency and should be corrected with scar lysis and middle lamellar augmentation. If the lid margin is elevated with superior traction on the lid, lateral traction should then be applied. If the ectropion corrects, the retraction may be caused by eyelid laxity and may be corrected with an eyelid tightening procedure such as a lateral tarsal strip. If the retraction improves with 2-finger elevation but does not correct with lateral tension on the lid, the disorder is likely caused by anterior lamella deficiency and can be corrected with anterior lamella augmentation (**Fig. 4**).

Entropion occurs when the lid margin turns posteriorly toward the globe. The lashes and keratinized skin rubbing against the eye can cause mechanical damage to the cornea and conjunctiva and can cause extreme pain and irritation. Entropion can be caused by cicatrix, but is most commonly caused by involutional change. Evaluation of an entropion can also be aided by the examination techniques described earlier. If the 2-finger test is applied and the lid margin elevates and the entropion improves with lateral tension on the lid, the entropion is likely involutional and can be corrected with a lid tightening procedure. If the lid remains retracted after the 2-finger test the entropion is likely caused by posterior and middle lamella deficiency and should be treated with scar lysis and lamella augmentation (see **Fig. 4**).

SURGICAL CORRECTION

Optimization of scar outcome is best done during the initial operation, whether it is repair of a traumatic or oncologic deformity. Prevention of unfavorable outcomes requires meticulous attention to reconstruction of anatomic layers, restoration

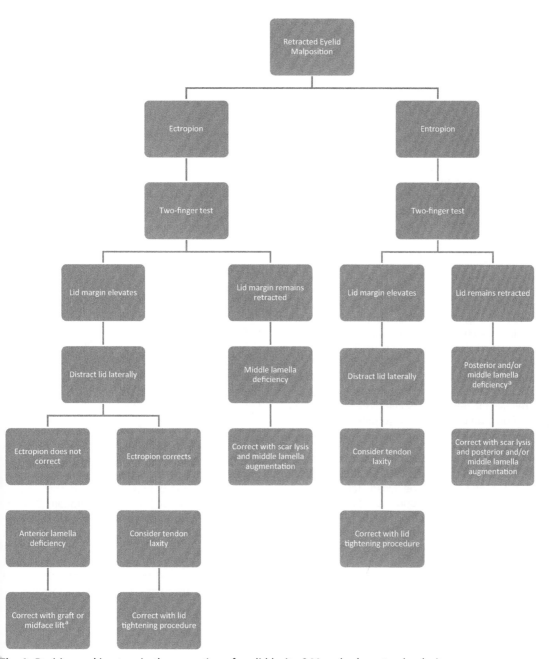

Fig. 4. Decision-making tree in the correction of eyelid laxity. [a] May also have tendon laxity.

of underlying support structures, and precise suturing technique with wound edge eversion as appropriate. Consideration can then be given to adjuvant postoperative therapies such as topical silicone gel or laser camouflage as described elsewhere in this issue.

For proper scar revision and retraction repair, the anterior and posterior lamella must be reconstructed separately. Once the disorder has been identified by proper examination techniques and

observation of lid movement, the malposition can be appropriately addressed. The anatomic function of each layer of the eyelid must be respected. The thin skin of the anterior lamella must be matched as closely as possible to allow the natural dynamic movement of the eyelid blink. Full-thickness skin graft options include the contralateral eyelid skin, posterior auricular skin, and supraclavicular skin. Graft donor sites should be free of hair, as well as evidence of malignancy, and care should be taken to ensure the closest color and texture match. Partial-thickness skin grafts have a high contraction rate and are not well suited for anterior lamellar grafting. The orbicularis should be preserved if possible to provide adequate closure and tonic tone of the eyelid.

The posterior lamella including the tarsus and conjunctiva should also be reconstructed if necessary. The tarsus provides structural support for the eyelid and is important to maintain stability of the eyelid margin. The conjunctiva provides a smooth mucosal surface that is in constant contact with the eye and is important to help prevent mechanical damage to the cornea and conjunctiva.

Cicatricial Retraction with Ectropion

Anterior lamellar shortening may be caused by trauma, overly aggressive lower eyelid blepharoplasty with skin removal, actinic changes, or after excision of eyelid malignancies. If the anterior lamella has been identified as insufficient by the 2-finger test, local flaps such as Z-plasties can be considered to direct tension horizontally instead of vertically. Elevation of the midface may also provide adequate anterior lamellar skin to resolve the retraction. Some regression of surgical effect can occur with these procedures.[8]

Anterior lamellar skin grafting is the gold standard for cicitrical ectropion.

1. A subciliary incision is marked after identifying the scar tissue to be lysed, taking care to extend the lysis beyond the cicatrix.
2. Local anesthetic with epinephrine is injected into the eyelid with a 30-gauge needle.
3. Place two 4.0 silk sutures into the lid margin to provide traction.
4. Make a subciliary incision with a number 15 Bard-Parker blade.
5. Use sharp dissection with Westcott scissors to lyse all scar tissue.
6. With the eyelid on traction with the silk sutures, mark a template for the full-thickness skin graft.
7. Harvest a full-thickness skin graft from the contralateral upper eyelid, supraclavicular skin, or posterior auricular skin.
8. Thin the graft, removing any subcuticular fat with scissors.
9. Suture the graft into place using 5.0 fast gut suture or 6.0 nylon suture and cover the graft with ophthalmic antibiotic ointment.
10. Tape the 4.0 traction silk sutures to the forehead to provide traction.
11. Tie a bolster over the graft with 4.0 silk sutures.
12. If there is any eyelid laxity, a lid tightening procedure such as a lateral tarsal strip should be performed. This procedure also provides tension during the healing process to decrease further cicatrix.

The bolster and traction sutures are removed after 1 week. The lid may appear overcorrected and the graft may be dark, but this typically resolves with healing. Massage is encouraged after 2 weeks.[9]

Cicatricial Retraction with Entropion

Posterior lamellar cicatrix can be caused by trauma, surgery, chemical injury, ocular cicatricial pemphigoid, Stevens-Johnson syndrome, trachoma, and chronic inflammation. If the cicatrix is caused by inflammatory disorders, ideally surgical intervention should be delayed until the disease is quiescent if possible.

There are many options for posterior lamellar spacing for correction of eyelid retraction and entropion. Free tarsus grafting from the contralateral upper eyelid is ideal because it is matched tissue and has conjunctival lining attached. Hard palate is considered to be an excellent option because of its structural rigidity and mucosal lining, although caution should be exercised because the hard palate mucosa is keratinized and can cause corneal irritation and damage.[10–12] Auricular cartilage can be effective because of its rigidity, but it can become lumpy and can be associated with eyelid thickening.[13] Xenografts (EnduraGen; Stryker Corporation, Newnan, GA) and Acellular dermis matrix allografts (AlloDerm; LifeCell Corporation, Branchburg, NJ) are associated with a high rate of retraction and resorption but are often used because a donor site is not needed.[14] Upper eyelid grafting is particularly important because it comes in contact with the cornea and the authors prefer free tarsal grafting from the contralateral eyelid if possible.

Cicatricial Retraction with Entropion: Correction with Free Tarsal Graft

Harvesting graft

1. Local anesthetic with epinephrine is injected into the pretarsal orbicularis on the contralateral upper eyelid of the recipient site (**Fig. 5**).
2. The eyelid is everted and the same local anesthetic is injected under the conjunctiva and Müller muscle.
3. The patient is prepped and draped.
4. A 4.0 silk suture is placed into the eyelid margin to provide traction and the eyelid is everted on Desmarres retractors.
5. Calipers are used to mark 4 mm above the eyelid margin and a line is drawn at this level

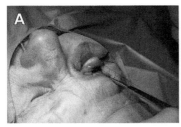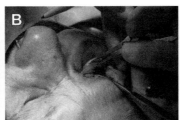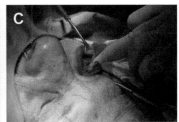

Fig. 5. Harvesting of a tarsal graft. (*A*) Eversion of the lid over a Desmarres retractor. (*B*) Measuring the graft size. (*C*) Donor defect after graft harvest left to heal by secondary intention.

parallel with the margin. This line is marked because 4 mm of tarsus should be left in the donor eyelid.

6. A number 15 Bard-Parker blade is used to incise the conjunctiva and tarsus along the line previously marked 4 mm above the eyelid margin. Take care not to go full thickness with this incision and preserve the overlying orbicularis muscle.

7. The 15 blade is then used to make vertical incisions superiorly along the conjunctiva and tarsus medially and laterally.

8. Careful dissection with blunt and sharp dissection using Westcott scissors is used to free the tarsal graft from the overlying orbicularis muscle.

9. Westcott scissors are used to cut the conjunctiva on the superior boarder of tarsus and remove the tarsal graft from the eyelid.

10. The tarsal graft is placed on the Mayo stand in a damp sponge until the donor site is prepared.

11. Remove the traction sutures and place the eyelid to its natural position. The graft donor site will reepithelialize and does not need to be closed.

Retraction repair and preparation of implant site

1. Local anesthetic with epinephrine is injected into the eyelid with a 30-gauge needle on the conjunctival side.

2. Place two 4.0 silk sutures into the lid margin to provide traction.

3. Incise the conjunctiva below the tarsal plate with a number 15 Bard-Parker blade, lysing the cicatricial bands with Westcott scissors.

4. Put tension on the silk traction sutures and using palpation feel for any remaining cicatrix.

5. If there is also scarring of the middle lamella, lyse this with sharp dissection. Avoid cautery if possible to decrease the chance of recurrent cicatrix.

6. Once the scar bands have been lysed and the lid can protract freely, suture the free conjunctival graft into place with the conjunctival side facing the fornix. Running 6.0 gut sutures can be used to secure the graft to the wound edges.

7. Tape the 4.0 traction silk sutures to the skin keeping the lid on stretch.

8. Tape the 4.0 traction silk sutures to the forehead to provide traction.

9. If there is any eyelid laxity, a lid tightening procedure, such as a lateral tarsal strip, should be performed. This procedure also provides tension during the healing process to decrease further cicatrix.

Remove the traction sutures at the 1-week postoperative visit and apply ophthalmic antibiotic ointment to the wound 3 times per day for 10 days.

Horizontal Tightening of the Eyelid

Lid tightening procedures play a role in eyelid stabilization for entropion as well as ectropion and help elevate the lid in cases of retraction. Canthopexy does not correct retraction caused by cicatrix unless the primary disorder has been appropriately addressed and the lid is mobilized. Use of the algorithm described earlier helps to direct treatment appropriately. The workhorse of eyelid surgeons is the lateral tarsal strip, which involves shortening the lower lid and reattaching it to the lateral orbital rim.[15] The lateral tarsal strip can be of significant value to support the lid when combined with the procedures to treat cicatricial ectropion and entropion described earlier.

For cases of advanced lateral canthal displacement in which simultaneous repositioning of the upper and lower limbs of the lateral retinaculum is desired, lateral transorbital canthopexy, as described elsewhere, can also be effective.[16]

Lateral tarsal strip procedure

1. Local anesthetic with epinephrine is injected into the lateral canthal area, infiltrating the

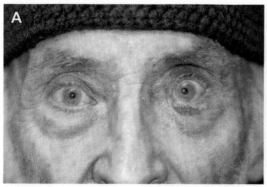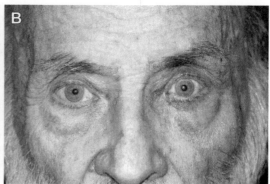

Fig. 6. Correction of the laterally displaced medial canthus. (*A*) Preoperative appearance after traumatic scarring of medial canthus. Note rounding and lateral displacement of the left medial canthus. (*B*) Appearance after correction with restoration of canthal symmetry.

lateral third of the lower lid and down to the orbital rim at the lateral canthus (**Fig. 3**).

2. A number 15 Bard-Parker blade is used to incise the skin at the lateral canthus, starting at the lateral canthal angle and continuing laterally for 0.5 to 1 cm.

3. Westcott scissors are used to make a lateral canthotomy, placing 1 blade into the fornix at the lateral canthal angle and 1 blade through the skin incision created.

4. Pick the lower eyelid up anteriorly with significant tension using Adson forceps. With Westcott scissors, strum the inferior crus of the lateral canthal tendon. Use scissors to cut the tendon and the lid should release from the rim.

5. Hemostasis is achieved at this point to decrease the chance of intraorbital hematoma formation.

6. The eyelid is pulled laterally and Westcott scissors are used to separate the anterior and posterior lamella between the tarsus and orbicularis muscle. Estimate the amount of lid shortening needed and dissect to that level; 5 mm is usually a good starting point.

7. Westcott scissors are used to cut the eyelid margin mucocutaneous junction away, leaving the superior border of tarsus exposed.

8. Westcott scissors are used to cut along the lower border of tarsus, removing the lower eyelid retractors.

9. A number 15 Bard-Parker blade is used to denude the conjunctival epithelium from the posterior border of tarsus.

10. The fashioned tarsal strip is pulled laterally to the periosteum to evaluate for appropriate tension. Westcott scissors can be used to conservatively shorten the strip if there is excess tarsus.

11. A 4.0 double-armed Mersilene suture on a P-2 needle is passed in a mattress fashion from posterior to anterior through the tarsal strip. The 2 ends of the suture are then passed through the periosteum at the level of the superior crus of the lateral canthal tendon and posterior into the orbit at the lateral orbital tubercle of Whitnall from posterior to anterior. A robust periosteal bite is made with both passes.

12. The suture is tied, the tarsal strip passes on the inner aspect of the rim, and the lid is directed posteriorly, keeping contact with the globe laterally. If there is space between the lid and the globe, the periosteal pass is not posterior enough and should be replaced.

13. Tension is checked and the lid should distract a few millimeters from the globe when pulled anteriorly.

14. The excess skin and orbicularis is trimmed including the eyelashes.

15. A 6.0 Vicryl suture is passed through the cut edge of the lower lid laterally and through the eyelid margin at the gray line. The suture is then passed through the gray line of the upper lid and out of the wound edge. The suture is tied to reapproximate the lateral canthal angle and close the canthotomy.

16. The lateral skin incision is closed with interrupted 6.0 gut sutures.[9,16]

Reconstruction of the medial canthal region

The medical canthus is challenging to reconstruct because it surrounds the lacrimal system. Although several procedures have been developed to tighten the anterior limb of the medial canthal tendon, increased tension in this anteromedial vector can pull the medial lid and canaliculi away from the globe. This problem can be

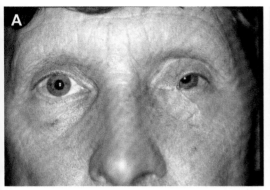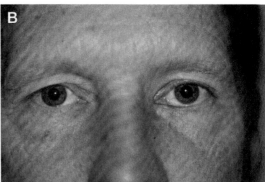

Fig. 7. Scarring of medial upper and lower eyelids in patient who underwent grafting after oncologic resection. (*A*) Preoperative appearance. The medial canthus has been obliterated with a graft extending vertically across, causing a marked visual field deficit. (*B*) Postoperative appearance after separation of the upper and lower lids, scar excision, and precaruncular medial canthopexy.

overcome by tightening the posterior limb of the medial canthal tendon using a precaruncular approach[17] to perform a precaruncular medial canthopexy.[18] This procedure can be used for cases of medial canthal dystopic caused by traumatic scarring (**Fig. 6**) or the correction of postoncologic reconstructive deformity (**Figs. 7 and 8**).

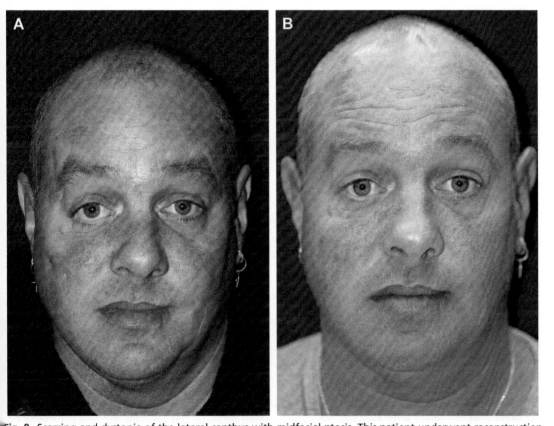

Fig. 8. Scarring and dystopia of the lateral canthus with midfacial ptosis. This patient underwent reconstruction of zygomaticomaxillary fractures, which included lateral canthotomy. The patient developed midface ptosis and rounding of the lateral canthus, which resulted in symptomatic ectropion (*A*). Lateral transorbital canthopexy was performed with lysis of cicatricial adhesions and endoscopic midface lift, correcting the deformity (*B*). Note the elevation of the lateral retinaculum with restoration of an acute angle between the upper and lower lateral eyelids and elevation of the malar fat pad.

1. Local anesthetic is injected as described earlier.
2. Probes are placed into the superior and inferior canaliculi for protection.
3. The caruncle is retracted laterally, and a Westcott scissor is used to incise between the conjunctiva and skin. This plane is opened by spreading the scissors, and the posterior limb of the medial canthal tendon, located at the medial border of the dissection, is followed to the posterior lacrimal crest. A permanent 4.0 suture is placed through the periorbital at the superior aspect of the lacrimal crest. The conjunctival incision is then extended laterally to incise the medial tarsus immediately lateral to the inferior canaliculus (to maintain patency of the canaliculus). The suture is then passed through the tarsus. The suture is then tied to provide the desired tension in the medial lid, and the knot is rotated into the orbit. Closure of the conjunctiva is generally not required.

Combining procedures

For complex eyelid malposition, it is common for several of the procedures described earlier to be required to correct the periorbital scarring and restore physiologic lid support. Performing lateral canthal tightening without strengthening the medial canthus can allow the lid to slide laterally, worsening the underlying condition. In these cases, it is optimal to first place the medial canthal sutures without tying them, then place the lateral canthal sutures. The tension in the medial and lateral sutures can then be adjusted to angle the lid appropriately. Once the appropriate tension is chosen, the medial sutures are tied off and then the lateral sutures are fixated. In these cases, ancillary procedures such as midface lift and anterior lamella grafting are performed as indicated (**Fig. 9**).

Nonsurgical intervention

Cicatricial retraction of the eyelid should be prevented if possible, by avoiding suturing or cauterizing the orbital septum when operating and avoiding vertical tension on the eyelid during periorbital reconstruction. Often the eyelid is in good position after trauma or periorbital surgery only to begin retraction in the postoperative period. Recently 5-fluorouacil (5-FU) has been shown to modulate scar formation after intralesional injection.[19–22] Intralesional steroid injection has been used for some time by many clinicians for modulation of scarring as well. 5-FU is an antimetabolite traditionally used for gastrointestinal, breast, and

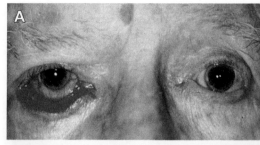

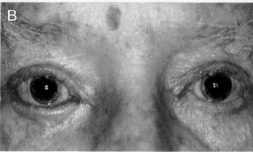

Fig. 9. Cicatricial ectropion. (*A*) Preoperative appearance. (*B*) After precaruncular medial canthopexy, lower lid anterior lamella grafting, transorbital lateral canthopexy, and bilateral brow lift. Note the elevation of the lateral canthus relative to the medial canthus.

ovarian cancers. It has been shown to break down hypertrophic scars presumably by reducing fibroblast proliferation as well as by inhibiting collagen type 1 production.[23] Type 1 collagen is found in high concentrations in scars and is thought to play an important role in scarring.[24] Intralesional 5-FU for scar modulation is an off-label use and should be avoided in patients with active chronic infections or immune depression, and in pregnant or lactating women.[25] 5-FU has significant adverse hematologic effects, such as anemia, thrombocytopenia, and leukopenia; however these are usually seen with intravenous dosing.[26] Shah and colleagues[27] did a comprehensive review of 5-FU for the treatment of hypertrophic scars and the most serious side effects included dehiscence, widened scar, and tissue necrosis; however, most studies reported no side effects from treatment. 5-FU combined with corticosteroids injected into scars has shown promising effects.[27] For periorbital scarring, Massry[28] reports improvement with periorbital cicatrix using a 1:3 mixture of Kenalog, 5 mg/mL, with 5-FU, 50 mg/mL, injected every 3 weeks for a total of 3 injections. A mixture of Kenalog and 5-FU injected into traumatic or postoperative eyelids with retraction caused by cicatrix should be considered as a nonsurgical option (**Fig. 10**).

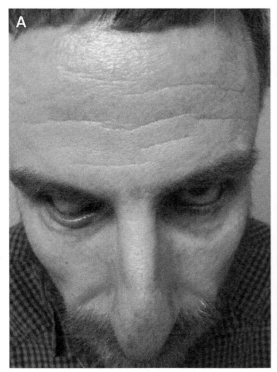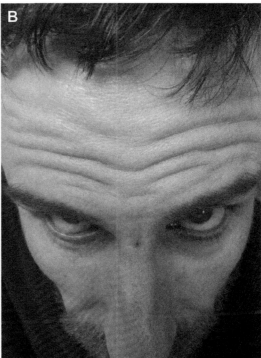

Fig. 10. Cicatricial ectropion right lower lid. (*A*) Before intervention. (*B*) One week after single injection of 5-FU/Kenalog. Note restoration of normal lid position, including the medial canthal region.

SUMMARY

Periorbital scarring with eyelid retraction can have serious visual effects and can lead to loss of vision or even loss of the eye. Understanding of eyelid anatomy and the delicate balance of its structural supports is critical for the identification of the eyelid disorder responsible for the cicatrix and helps to guide treatment. The 2-finger test and lateral distraction of the lid can also be of significant help in proper diagnosis of the underlying disorder. Proper reconstruction with respect to the anterior and posterior lamellae helps to ensure a favorable outcome.

REFERENCES

1. Ridgeway JM, Larrabee WF. Anatomy for blepharoplasty and brow-lift. Facial Plast Surg 2010;26(3): 177–85.
2. Goold LA, Casson RJ, Selva D, et al. Tarsal height [Letter to the editor]. Ophthalmology 2009;116:1831.
3. Dutton J. Atlas of clinical and surgical orbital anatomy. 2nd edition. Philadelphia: Elsevier Saunders; 2011. p. 141.
4. Anderson RL. The medial canthal tendon branches out. Arch Ophthalmol 1977;95:2051.
5. Ahl NC, Hill JD. Horner's muscle and the lacrimal system. Arch Ophthalmol 1982;100:488.
6. Jones LT. The anatomy of the lower eyelid and its relations to the cause and cure of ectropion. Am J Ophthalmol 1960;49:29.
7. Branham G, Holds JB. Brow/upper lid anatomy, aging and aesthetic analysis. Facial Plast Surg Clin North AM 2015;23(2):117–27.
8. Couch S, Custer P. Ectropion. In: Black EH, Nesi FA, Gladstone G, et al, editors. Smith and Nesi's Ophthalmic plastic and reconstructive surgery. 3rd edition. New York: Springer; 2012. p. 329.
9. Nerad J. Treatment of ectropion. In: Techniques in ophthalmic plastic surgery. Amsterdam: Elsevier; 2010. p. 81–97.
10. Wearne MJ, Sandy C, Rose GE, et al. Autogenous hard palate mucosa: the ideal lower eyelid spacer. Br J Ophthalmol 2001;85:1183–7.
11. Feorgescu D, Belsare G, McCann JD, et al. Management of the post-lower eyelid blepharoplasty retracted eyelid. In: Massry GG, Murphy MR, Azizzadeh B, editors. Master techniques in blepharoplasty and periorbital rejuvenation. New York: Springer; 2011. p. 199–210.
12. Chandra S. Text book of dental and oral histology with embryology. 2nd edition. New Delhi (India): Jaypee Brothers' Medical Publishing; 2002. p. 176.

13. Obear MF, Smith B. Tarsal grafting to elevate the lower lid margin. Am J Ophthalmol 1965;59:1088–90.

14. Sullivan SA, Dailey RA. Graft contraction: a comparison of acellular dermis versus hard palate mucosa in lower eyelid surgery. Ophthal Plast Reconstr Surg 2003;19:14–24.

15. Anderson RL, Gordy DD. The tarsal strip procedure. Arch Ophthalmol 1979;97:2192–6.

16. Moe KS, Linder T. Lateral transorbital canthopexy. JAMA Facial Plast Surg 2000;2(1):9–15.

17. Moe KS. The precaruncular approach to the medial orbit. JAMA Facial Plast Surg 2003;5(6):483–7.

18. Moe KS, Kao CH. Precaruncular medial canthopexy. JAMA Facial Plast Surg 2005;7(4):244–50.

19. Berman B, Viera MH, Amini S, et al. Prevention and management of hypertrophic scars and keloids after burns in children. J Craniofac Surg 2008;19: 989–1006.

20. Fitzpatrick RE. Treatment of inflamed hypertrophic scars using intralesional 5-FU. Dermatol Surg 1999;25:224–32.

21. Gupta S, Karla A. Efficacy and safety of intralesional 5-fluorouacil in the treatment of keloids. Dermatology 2002;204:130–2.

22. Yoo DB, Azizzadeh B, Massry GG. Injectable 5-FU with or without added steroid in periorbital skin grafting: initial observations. Ophthal Plast Reconstr Surg 2015;31:122–6.

23. Khaw PT, Sherwood MB, MacKay SL, et al. Five-minute treatments with fluorouracil, floxuridine, and mitomycin have long-term effects on human Tenon's capsule fibroblasts. Arch Ophthalmol 1992;110:1150–4.

24. Occleston NL, Daniels JT, Tarnuzzer RW, et al. Single exposures to antiproliferatives: long-term effects on ocular fibroblast wound healing behavior. Invest Ophthalmol Vis Sci 1997;38:1998–2007.

25. Gold MG, McGuire M, Mustoe TA, et al. Updated international clinical recommendation on scar management: part 2 algorithms for scar prevention and treatment. Dermatol Surg 2014;40(8):825–31.

26. Uppal RS, Khan U, Kakar S, et al. The effects of a single dose of 5-fluorouracil on keloid scars: a clinical trial of timed wound irrigation after extralesional excision. Plast Reconstr Surg 2001;105(5): 1218–24.

27. Shah VV, Aldahan AS, Mlacker S, et al. 5-Fluorouracil in the treatment of keloids and hypertrophic scars: a comprehensive review of the literature. Dermatol Ther 2016;6:169–83.

28. Massry GG. Cicatricial canthal webs. Ophthal Plast Reconstr Surg 2011;27(6):426–30.

Treating Scars of the Cheek Region

CrossMark

Kofi Derek Boahene, MD[a],*, James A. Owusu, MD[b]

KEYWORDS

- Cheek scar • Scar camouflage • Non-surgical scar revision

KEY POINTS

- Scars of the cheek resulting from all causes can extol significant psychological toll.
- The cheek is the largest facial subunit and is visually and aesthetically prominent, making scars in this region difficult to ignore.
- An approach to scar management that targets specific characteristics of a scar using a combination of surgical and nonsurgical modalities can significantly improve the appearance of most scars.
- The ideal time to revise a scar should be based on the extent of scar maturation and presence or absence of any functional distortion.

INTRODUCTION

In times past, scars on the cheek were worn as badges of honor; signs of battle hardiness or prowess in duels. These so-called good scars were worn in a fashionable manner and did not invite negative stares. In contrast, scars resulting from traumatic events such as an assault, a dog bite, acne, or cancer treatment can have a life-long psychological impact that is more than skin deep. Studies using eye tracking have shown that the eye, nose, and lip form the central triangle of visual fixation the primary focus of most face-to-face interactions. This normal pattern of visual scan path changes significantly with attentional bias to the cheek when scars are present.[1] The goal of scar revision is to efface the visual characteristics that attracts negative evaluation by observers and mend the adverse psychological imprints that surrounds the cause and living with the scar. An objective measure of a successful cheek scar revision will be normalization of pretreatment visual scan paths and an associated improvement in self-confidence.

In general, scars can be effaced and camouflaged but not made to vanish completely. Effacement and camouflaging are visual concepts that play on the properties of light absorption and reflection. It is therefore important to understand the physical features of a scar and their effect on visual perception when outlining a plan for scar revision. Similarly, the surface anatomy of the cheek subunits, the texture of the skin, and the underling volumetric and contour changes should be considered in treatment regimens to create a favorable cheek scar.

ANATOMIC CONSIDERATIONS

The cheek is the largest aesthetic facial subunit extending from the zygomatic arch and orbital crease superiorly to the lower border of the mandible inferiorly. Medially, the cheek is bordered by the nasofacial sulcus, and nasolabial

Financial Disclosure: None.

Conflicts of Interest: None.

[a] Department of Otorhinolaryngology, The Johns Hopkins Hospital, 601 N Caroline Street, Baltimore, MD 48109, USA; [b] Department of Otorhinolaryngology – Head and Neck Surgery, University of Texas Health Sciences Center at Houston, 6400 Fannin Street, Houston, TX 77030, USA

* Corresponding author.

E-mail address: dboahen1@jhmi.edu

facialplastic.theclinics.com

and nasomandibular creases, and extends to the preauricular crease laterally. Based on the underlying bony skeleton and soft tissue coverage, the cheek subunit is further divided into infraorbital, zygomatic, nasolabial, buccal, and parotidomasseteric (preauricular) anatomic subunits. The thickness of the skin coverage varies across the anatomic subunits of the cheek. Skin of the infraorbital subunit is particularly thin as it transitions onto the lower eyelid. The zygomatic subunit overlies the zygomatic arch and malar prominence; the skin in this region has minimal laxity; it is fixed to the underlying fascia. The topography of the cheek transitions from a convex zygomatic subunit to a flat buccal subunit. The skin of the buccal subunit is thicker than that of the other subunits and is freely mobile over the underlying subcutaneous tissue and fascia. The parotidomasseteric subunit is the region overlying the parotid gland. The skin in this region is thinner and relatively fixed compared with that of the buccal subunit. The skin in the nasolabial subunit is thick and mobile, similar to that of the buccal subunit. The nasolabial crease is formed by direct attachment of dermis to the underlying muscles (levator labii superioris alaeque nasi and orbicularis oris) owing to the absence of the superficial musculoaponeurotic system in this area.[2] The orientation of collagen fibers and action of the underlying muscles create relaxed skin tension lines (RSTLs) on the cheek that are curvilinear, running from the malar eminence to the inferior border of the mandible (**Fig. 1**). Cutaneous perforators from the infraorbital, transverse facial, angular, and zygomaticofacial arteries supply the skin of the cheek.

EVALUATING A PATIENT CHEEK SCAR FOR REVISION

A detailed history of how a scar was acquired and an outline of any previous treatment are important when assessing a patient for scar revision. For example, traumatic scars allowed to heal by secondary intention may leave broad and poorly textured scars that are likely to respond well to controlled surgical repair. In contrast, a scar that has failed to improve by reexcision by an experienced surgeon may need to be approached differently because another excision is unlikely to yield significant improvement. Medical comorbidities, as far as they influence wound healing, should be considered when assessing scars for revision. A history of poor wound healing and systemic disease such as diabetes can affect the outcome of scar revision. Although individuals with darker skin tones are more prone to developing hypertrophic scarring, a patient-specific wound healing

history may be more informative than a generalized skin type categorization.[3,4]

The features of a scar that make it visually perceptible can direct the design and selection of a treatment modality for improving cheek scars. Cheek scars should be assessed for their color match with surrounding skin, vascularity, light reflection, texture, contour, pliability, height, relation to the RSTLs, and any distortion of the eyelid, lip, or nasal alar (**Fig. 2**).

A wide scar may be improved by narrowing; a depressed scar that absorbs light resulting in a visible shadow is best corrected by addressing the contour discrepancy. Scars that are thick and raised may be flattened with either surgical or nonsurgical techniques and those with color and texture mismatch may be addressed with modalities that improve color and texture blend. A favorable scar is parallel to RSTLs or is hidden along the borders of aesthetic subunits. Thus, misaligned scars may be broken up and reoriented to more closely match RSTLs or repositioned into aesthetic subunit boundaries. Although preplanned surgical incisions may be placed in RSTLs, traumatic scars do not necessary respect these anatomic boundaries and may require reorienting techniques for better camouflage.

TIMING OF SCAR REVISION

Most scars improve with time; therefore, ample time should be allowed for healing and scar maturation before any major revision is considered.[3,5] The process of scar maturation seems to be faster in patients older than 55 years old when compared with patients younger than 30 years old. The clinical macroscopic appearance of the scar, particularly the presence and progression of redness, correlates well with extent of scar maturation.[6] Together with the patients' age, the macroscopic appearance may be used to anticipate and plan the timing of any interventions. Scars that may be improved by resurfacing techniques may be treated early (6–8 weeks) in the wound healing process where the redness from the early inflammation is blended with that of the resurfacing process. Cheek scars that cause retraction or distortion of the lower eyelid, nostril, or lip are likely to worsen with scar maturation and can be revised early.

CHEEK SCAR REVISION TECHNIQUES

Several surgical and nonsurgical techniques are available for improving the appearance of cheek scars. The technique selected depends on the attribute of the scar that needs to be improved.

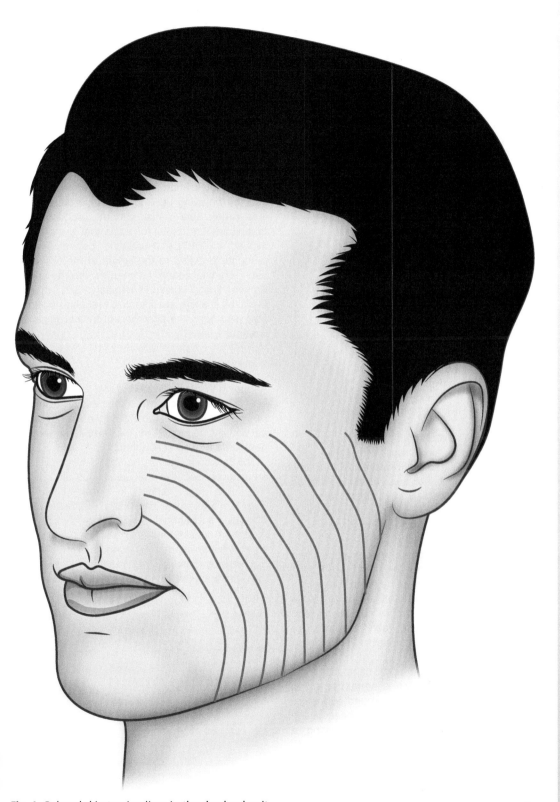

Fig. 1. Relaxed skin tension lines in the cheek subunit.

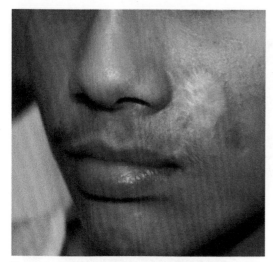

Fig. 2. Left cheek scar showing several unfavorable features that make a scar visually apparent. The scar is wide, hypopigmented, has a shiny surface, and interrupts aesthetic units (upper lip).

Compared with other facial subunits, the cheek has ample skin and most scars in this region can be revised using surrounding tissue.

EXCISION

Scars that have several undesirable features that cannot be improved significantly with a single modality are best excised and replaced with a new, more favorable scar. Excision can be performed as a single procedure or in multiple stages when the scar is too large to allow primary closure of the defect. Scar excision can be used to improve scars that are wide, atrophic, hypertrophic, depressed, or malpositioned. Wide scars that are parallel to RSTLs can be excised and closed using appropriate techniques to reduce tension on the closure. Unfavorable scars that are close to the boundary of the aesthetic unit may be excised and placed in a more favorable position. For example, scars in close proximity to the preauricular crease may be excised and repositioned in the preauricular crease for better camouflage. An elliptical or fusiform excision is performed along the margin of the scar and the wound edges are undermined to reduce tension. The base of the scar may be preserved to avoid creating a depressed scar. A layered closure is performed to reduce tension on the skin. Hypertrophic scars and keloids may benefit from intramarginal excision to decrease the risk of recurrence.[7] Owing to its large surface area, most scars on the cheek can be excised and closed primarily. Scars that are too large to permit primary closure can be excised in multiple stages 6 to 8 weeks apart (serial excision). An alternative to serial excision is tissue expansion. A tissue expander is placed adjacent to the scar and expanded over a time period to provide an adequate amount of skin to completely excise and replace the scar. Tissue expansion is useful when a large portion of the cheek needs to be replaced, which can occur in burn scars.[8]

SCAR IRREGULARIZATION

Scar irregularization improves the appearance of scar by breaking up a long, straight scar into a less predictable visual pattern. Irregularization techniques are useful for scars that are properly aligned to RSTLs or subunit boundaries but perceptible owing to the length of the scar. The main irregularization techniques are geometric broken lines, running W-plasty and running Z-plasty. Z-plasty in addition to irregularizing scars also lengthens the scar based on the angle between the flaps.

RUNNING W-PLASTY

A running W-plasty is used mainly to irregularize a linear curvilinear scar without increasing its length. Because of its predictable zigzag pattern, it is not as visually deceptive as the irregularly irregular geometric broken configuration.

The basic design of the W-plasty consists of creating consecutive triangular flaps along each side of a scar planned to perfectly interlock (**Fig. 3**). To minimize its visibility, each side of the triangular flap should not be more than 6 mm. Important considerations in designing a W-pasty on curvilinear scars is to account for the length discrepancy between the 2 sides by designing the outer triangles slightly larger in both side length

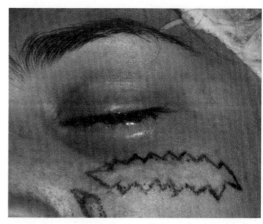

Fig. 3. A running W-plasty technique for irregularization of a cheek scar.

and angle than their counterparts on the inner curve. The deeper aspect of the scar may be preserved to create a stable base on which the new scar is formed. The preserved base also reduces the risk of forming a depressed scar. Running W-plasty does not redirect the final scar because there is no transposition of the triangular flaps. Therefore, to achieve a more favorable orientation, each triangle in the W may be modified from the classic design and oriented to more closely align with the RSTLs.

GEOMETRIC BROKEN LINES CLOSURE

Geometric broken line uses irregulary irregular patterns of scar excision using geometric figures with a width of 5 to 7 mm. The irregular pattern makes the resulting scar less predictable to the eye compared with a W-plasty. Considered a variant of the basic W-plasty, geometric broken lines closure does not lengthen the original scar. The design of the geometric broken lines closure follows from a pattern of irregular configuration of squares, rectangles, and triangles that are interlocked into complimentary shapes on either side of the scar. A useful approach to planning and constructing a geometric broken lines closure is to first fashion corresponding perpendicular lines 3 to 6 mm apart across the scar into which corresponding geometric shapes are designed to interlock perfectly (**Fig. 4**). As with the running W-plasty, the deep scar tissue may be preserved to act as an autofiller to minimize indentation of the final scar.

SCAR REPOSITIONING

Scars that are misaligned with RSTLs and subunit boundaries are usually visible to the observer. For better camouflage, misaligned scars may be repositioned to become more favorably oriented. Scars close to the preauricular crease can be repositioned in the crease, providing better camouflage. Repositioning may require removing intervening normal skin between the scar and the desired location. The nasolabial and infraorbital creases are

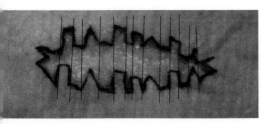

Fig. 4. Planning a scar revision with geometric broken line closure technique.

major landmarks on the cheek. Scars that interrupt these creases are usually unsightly and require repositioning. An improperly positioned scar in the infraorbital crease can also cause ectropion from retraction of the lower eyelid. A Z-plasty is a useful technique for realigning distorted landmarks. It also lengthens contracted scars and provides some irregularization. The degree of lengthening is dependent on the angles used to design the flaps. Classic Z-plasty involves transposition of 60° equilateral triangles that lengthens the scar by 75%. Triangles that are either 30° or 45° lengthen the scar by 25% and 50%, respectively. The scar is designed as the central limb of the "Z" and the orientation changes by 90°, 60°, and 45° for a 60°, 45°, and 30° Z-plasty, respectively.[9]

SUBSCISION

Subscision improves the appearance of depressed scars by releasing the tethered dermis to allow ingrowth of scar tissue to fill in the depression. This technique is particularly useful for treating depressed acne scars common on the cheek.[10] It involves the use of a needle to release the depressed dermis from the underlying tissue; the space created allows ingrowth of scar tissue lifting up the dermis. This can be combined with injection of filler or fat to fill the depression.

SCAR RESURFACING

Resurfacing can improve the texture and contour of a scar. Resurfacing can be performed using dermabrasion or a laser. Dermabrasion uses controlled abrasion of the skin down to the depth of the papillary to superficial reticular dermis to improve scar appearance. The depth of the papillary dermis is characterized by pinpoint bleeding; parallel white lines characterize the superficial reticular dermis. Abrasion deep into the reticular dermis may lead to worsening of the scar's appearance. Dermabrasion is best performed when fibroblast activity is high after allowing 6 to 8 weeks of wound healing. Scar improvement is achieved by increasing collagen organization.[11–13] Dermabrasion is a useful technique for improving acne scars, and early postoperative and traumatic scars. Periprocedural antivirals reduce the risk of herpetic outbreak. Isotretinoin causes apoptosis of pilosebaceous units that are responsible for regenerating the skin after dermabrasion and its use is a contraindication for dermabrasion.

LASER SCAR RESURFACING

Both ablative and nonablative lasers can be used to improve the appearance of scars. Ablative lasers improve scar appearance by ablating water-containing tissue in the superficial layer of the skin resulting deepithelialization and epidermal regeneration. There is also reorientation of collagen fibers in a mechanism similar to that of dermabrasion. The ablative lasers commonly used in scar revision are CO_2 and erbium:YAG. Both lasers cause superficial ablation, resulting in deepithelialization. CO_2 has a deeper depth of penetration compared with erbium:YAG and is associated with a longer recovery time. Fractional ablative laser resurfacing is an alternative method of resurfacing. The laser beam is delivered in a pixelated fashion, leaving areas of the skin untreated. There is faster regeneration of the treated areas from the intact skin. Ablative laser can be helpful in the treatment of hypertrophic, atrophic, and acne scars.[14–16] Similar to dermabrasion, periprocedural antivirals should be considered to help reduce the risk of herpetic outbreak.

Nonablative lasers create dermal injury to the dermis leaving the epidermis intact. It has moderate improvement of scars with minimal side effects compared with ablative lasers. The most widely used nonablative laser is the Nd:YAG. Studies report a 40% to 50% improvement in the appearance of atrophic scars with Nd:YAG treatment.[14] Pulsed dye laser is a nonablative laser with a hemoglobin chromophore. It is traditionally used in the treatment of vascular lesion. Pulsed dye laser can be used to improve scars with persistent erythema. It also improves contour and texture of hypertrophic scars.[14,17]

NONSURGICAL TECHNIQUES
Steroids and 5-Flourouracil

Injection of steroids can improve the appearance of hypertrophic scars, keloids, and scars with trapdoor deformity.[18] The most common form used is injectable triamcinolone acetonide (Kenalog; Delcor Asset Corp, Lake Forest, IL) in concentrations between 10 to 40 mg/mL. Topical steroids maybe used to diminish erythema 2 to 3 weeks after skin resurfacing. Dermal and subcutaneous atrophy may occur if an excess amount of steroid is used.

5-Fluoracil may be injected as an alternative to triamcinolone. 5-Fluoracil should be avoided when there is evidence of bone marrow suppression, including anemia, leukopenia, thrombocytopenia, and during pregnancy. Adverse effects of 5-fluoracil are generally limited to the injection site and include pain hyperpigmentation and skin irritation.

Autologous Platelet-Rich Plasma

Platelet-rich plasma is a highly concentrated autologous solution of plasma prepared from a patient's own blood. Platelet-rich plasma contains platelets that are alleged to release numerous growth factors that may be valuable in wound healing. Platelet-rich plasma has been used in combination with other scar treatment modalities such as microneedling and laser resurfacing to improve scars, including acne scars.

Silicone Sheets and Gels

Silicone sheets and gels may be used alone or in combination with other techniques to improve the appearance of hypertrophic scars and keloids. The exact mechanism of improvement is unknown, but is believed to be partially owing to increased hydration of the scar.

Mechanical Force

Massage of scars after complete epithelialization decreases adherence to deeper structures and improves the appearance.

Cosmetics

Cosmetics can conceal scars using a foundation or diminish the appearance of scars using color theory. Color theory uses opposite shades of a color to tone down its appearance. For example, a red scar is camouflage with green concealer, blue or purple scar with yellow concealer, and brown and yellow tones are neutralized with purple concealer.[19]

ACNE SCARS OF THE CHEEK

Acne scars occurring on the cheek are among the most common reasons patients seek facial scar revision. Treatment of acne scars incorporates almost all the modalities described herein, including surgical, nonsurgical, and the use of cosmoceuticals. There is no single treatment approach that works for all acne scars, but a regimen that combines preventative measures, active management, and maintenance protocols can be effective. Female patients who tend to have acne flare ups coincident with their menstrual cycle may be placed on prophylactic low-dose antibiotics for several cycles. They may be supplemented with topical antimicrobials and topical retinoids. In severe cases, isotretinoin has been found to be effective but must be instituted under close supervision. Acne scars are often depressed as a result of the secondary contraction from the associated inflammation. Deeply depressed and isolated scars may be punched out and closed. The resulting suture scars are usually flat and may be improved further by resurfacing. Diffuse and shallow acne scars may be improve with resurfacing techniques, microneedling, rolling, and subcision, as well as with fillers and laser application. Hypertrophic scars may be treated with triamcinolone injection. Hyperpigmentation is a common postinflammatory change seen in acne patients. Hyperpigmentation may be treated with skin-lightening topical creams such as hydroquinone, kojic acid, retinoids, or a superficial depth chemical peel.

SUMMARY

Scars of the cheek resulting from all causes can extol significant psychological toll. The cheek is the largest facial subunit and visually and aesthetically prominent making scars in this region difficult to ignore. An approach to scar management that targets specific characteristics of a scar using a combination of surgical and nonsurgical modalities can significantly improve the appearance of most scars. The ideal time to revise a scar should be based on the extent of scar maturation and presence or absence of any functional distortion.

REFERENCES

1. Ishii L, Carey J, Byrne P, et al. Measuring attentional bias to peripheral facial deformities. Laryngoscope 2009;119(3):459–65.
2. Gassner HG, Rafii A, Young A, et al. Surgical anatomy of the face: implications for modern facelift techniques. Arch Facial Plast Surg 2008;10(1):9–19.
3. Schweinfurth JM, Fedok F. Avoiding pitfalls and unfavorable outcomes in scar revision. Facial Plast Surg 2001;17:273–8.
4. Visscher MO, Bailey JK, Hom DB. Scar treatment variations by skin type. Facial Plast Surg Clin North Am 2014;22(3):453–62.
5. Shockley WW. Scar revision techniques: z-plasty, w-plasty, and geometric broken line closure. Facial Plast Surg Clin North Am 2011;19(3):455–63.
6. Bond JS, Duncan JA, Sattar A, et al. Maturation of human scar : an observational study. Plast Reconstr Surg 2008;121(5):1650–8.
7. Engrave LH, Gottlieb JR, Millard SP, et al. A comparison of intramarginal and extramarginal excision of hypertrophic burn scars. Plast Reconstr Surg 1988;81:40–5.
8. Spence RJ. Expanded transposition flap technique for total and subtotal resurfacing of the face and neck. J Burns Wounds 2007;6:e8.
9. Thomas JR, Prendiville S. Update in scar revision. Facial Plast Surg Clin North Am 2002;10:103–11.
10. Orentreich DS, Orentreich N. Subcutaneous incisionless (subcision) surgery for the correction of depressed scars and wrinkles. Dermatol Surg 1995;21:543–9.
11. Harmon CB, Zelickson BD, Roenigk RK, et al. Dermabrasive scar revision. Immunohistochemical and ultrastructural evaluation. Dermatol Surg 1995; 21(6):503–8.
12. Katz BE, Oca AG. A controlled study of the effectiveness of spot dermabrasion ('scarabrasion') on the appearance of surgical scars. J Am Acad Dermatol 1991;24:462–6.
13. Surowitz JB, Shockley WW. Enhancement of facial scars with dermabrasion. Facial Plast Surg Clin North Am 2011;19:517–25.
14. Oliaei S, Nelson JS, Fitzpatrick R, et al. Use of lasers in acute management of surgical and traumatic incisions on the face. Facial Plast Surg Clin North Am 2011;19:543–50.
15. Khatri KA, Mahoney DL, McCartney MJ. Laser scar revision: a review. J Cosmet Laser Ther 2011; 13(2):54–62.
16. Tanzi EL, Alster TS. Comparison of a 1450nm diode laser and a 1320nm Nd:YAG laser in the treatment of atrophic facial scars: a prospective clinical and histologic study. Dermatol Surg 2004;30:152–7.
17. Oliaei S, Nelson JS, Fitzpatrick R, et al. Laser treatment of scars. Facial Plast Surg 2012;28(5):518–24.
18. Moran ML. Scar revision. Otolaryngol Clin North Am 2001;34:767–80.
19. Sidle DM, Decker JR. Use of makeup, hairstyles, glasses, and prosthetics as adjuncts to scar camouflage. Facial Plast Surg Clin North Am 2011;19: 481–9.

Unique Clinical Aspects of Nasal Scarring

Benjamin P. Caughlin, MD[a,b], Christian Barnes, MD[a], J. Stuart Nelson, MD, PhD[a], Brian J.F. Wong, MD, PhD[a,*]

KEYWORDS

- Scar revision • Laser • Nasal scar • Facial scar • Surgical scar revision

KEY POINTS

- Various methods are available for refining scars of the external nose and optimal scar revision frequently requires the utilization of multiple techniques.
- Differing anatomy of nasal subunits and their underlying structural framework limit surgical options in nasal scar revision compared with other areas of the face.
- An understanding of a variety of laser technologies and their specific applications can vastly aid in fine, controlled scar revision.
- Achieving optimal scar reduction regularly requires multiple stages of intervention, close follow-up, and repeat procedures.

A main focus of facial aesthetic surgery is to draw attention to the eyes. Any imperfection in nasal contour that leads to asymmetry will be noticed, and this emphasizes the importance of treating nasal injury and scar formation aggressively. The flexible cartilaginous framework of the nose is enveloped by a skin soft tissue envelope (SSTE) of variable thickness. It is this framework particularly over the nasal tip that must counter the forces generated by wound healing and contracture. In contrast, over the superior nasal dorsum (supported by bone), and the middle vault (by the relatively firm fusion of the dorsal quadrangular and upper lateral cartilages) deformation of the SSTE is less dramatic after injury or defect closure. The varying thickness of the skin in combination with the varying stability of the structural framework (eg, tip vs dorsum) leads to differences in response in contrast to scar and injury management in most other regions of the face. This is amplified by the ability of the eye to discern even small changes in facial symmetry and structure. For example, the smallest amount of contracture at the alar rim or soft tissue triangle can result in asymmetry and thus noticeable deformation. In contrast, injury and subsequent scar formation over the osseous nasal framework can be treated conservatively, as the surface is firm and adjacent skin is linked to bone via periosteal attachments.

Finally, the nose is a functional organ that supports air flow and mechanically filters, warms, and humidifies inspired air. Significant scarring can lead to collapse of the internal and external nasal valves. All nasal surgeons must appreciate this when planning wound management or reconstruction and when deciding how to best treat nasal scars and defects.

MANAGEMENT AND TREATMENT
The Art of Doing Nothing

Healing by secondary intention can produce stable outcomes that are cosmetically acceptable, when applied in a measured and judicious manner. This is important to consider especially

[a] UC Irvine Department of Head & Neck Surgery, 101 The City Drive South, Orange, CA 92868, USA; [b] Facial Plastic and Reconstructive Surgery, 50 E Washington, Chicago, IL 60602, USA
* Corresponding author.
E-mail address: bjwong@uci.edu

Facial Plast Surg Clin N Am 25 (2017) 45–54
http://dx.doi.org/10.1016/j.fsc.2016.08.004
1064-7406/17/© 2016 Elsevier Inc. All rights reserved.

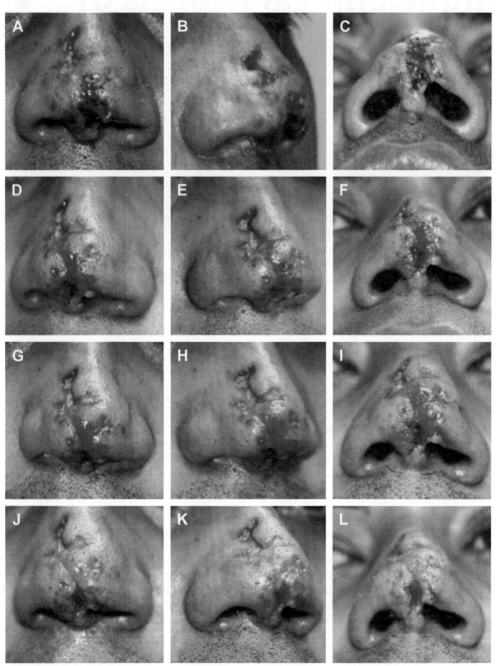

Fig. 1. The nasal tip of a 28-year-old Hispanic man who underwent open rhinoplasty with defatting of the tip SSTE and aggressive postoperative tape application (elsewhere). This led to postoperative vascular compromise followed by infection and tissue breakdown. The wound was treated with local wound care including antibiotic ointment (mupirocin) and frequent dressing changes during the acute phases of wound healing by the senior author (BJFW). The patient additionally received 6 rounds of hyperbaric oxygen therapy, frequent visits for wound debridement, comedone extractions, and 1 episode of free hand microneedling to release the scar. Images were obtained at presentation (A–C), 5 days (D–F), 1 week (G–I), 2 weeks (J–L), 4 weeks (M–O), 8 weeks (P–R), 14 weeks (S–U), and 27 weeks (V–X). The final images show the defect at 46 weeks and after 1 treatment with injectable hyaluronic acid (Y–AA) (performed elsewhere).

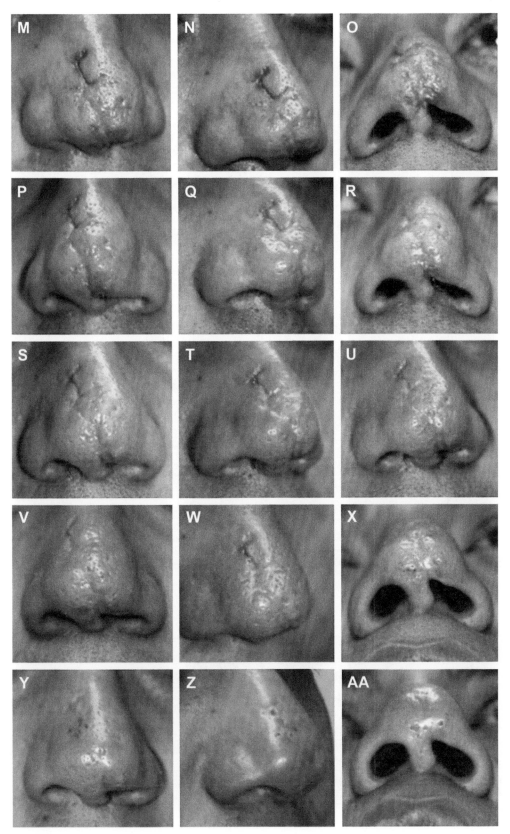

Fig. 1. (*continued*)

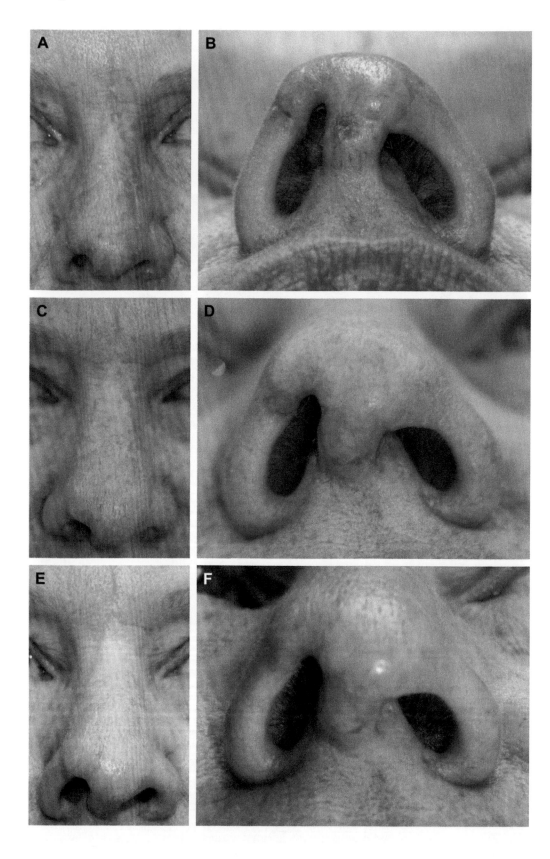

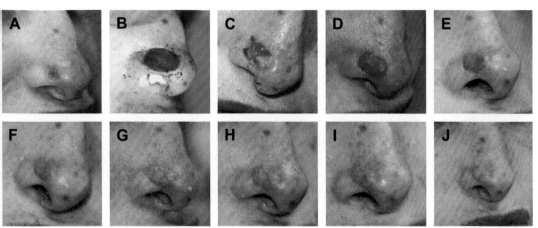

Fig. 3. A 44-year-old woman presents with morpheaform basal cell carcinoma of the right nasal ala (*A*). (*B*) Final defect after wide local excision of tumor. Surgical defect was covered with a hydrophilic dressing (MeroGel, Medtronic Xomed, Inc., Minneapolis, MN). Two weeks later, after pathologic confirmation of clear margins on permanent sections, the patient was taken back to the operating room for reconstruction with postauricular FTSG. The lesion as seen immediately before grafting (*C*) and 4 weeks after FTSG placement (*D*). The patient elected for no further treatment of the graft such as dermabrasion or laser resurfacing. Follow-up at 4 months (*E*), 10 months (*F*), 14 months (*G*), 23 months (*H*), 35 months (*I*), and 45 months after placement of skin graft (*J*).

with early scars produced by thermal injury or ballistic trauma in which the true extent of injury evolves over time. Aggressive local wound care is important, and this can be time and labor intensive, requiring frequent office visits and constant patient reassurance. The key is to strike a balance between doing the least-invasive treatment possible and obtaining the best results (**Fig. 1**). As no reconstructive surgery is performed, injury to normal adjacent tissue is minimized and other treatment options are preserved for future reconstruction if required. Adjunctive therapies, such as hyperbaric therapy,[1] local steroid injections,[2] silicone dressings,[3] massage,[4] pulsed dye laser,[5] fractionated laser,[6] and microneedling[7] may have value for modulating the evolving scar process. This works best over a concave surface overlying a firm bony framework, such as in the nasal dorsum adjacent to the canthal region.

Laser and Resurfacing

In our practice, the laser has largely replaced dermabrasion. Although many surgeons achieve outstanding results with dermabrasion, we focus on laser resurfacing for this section. The risk of laser devices to both physician and patient must be appreciated, and proper eye protection is imperative. A comprehensive understanding of the physiology of laser treatments for scars is evolving as technology advancement exceeds the rate of clinical adoption and use. In our practice, laser technology is used both early and later in treatment protocols.[8,9] We often start scar treatments with laser resurfacing and remodeling to varying degrees. This timing then allows us to better define the scar, to soften it, and to build the local collagen and tissues for any future reconstructions. If surgical scar revision is required, the reconstruction is followed again

Fig. 2. A 55-year-old woman with a history of melanoma in situ of the nasal dorsum resected by Mohs micrographic surgery (MMS) and reconstructed with nasal dorsum (Rieger) flap 8 months before presentation; note glabellar, dorsal, and sidewall scarring (*A*) (cancer resection and primary reconstruction performed elsewhere). Her recovery was complicated by wound infection that resolved with oral antibiotics. The patient used silicone strips to reduce scarring postoperatively and noted increased rotation of the tip with flap contracture (*A*). Unfortunately, she developed recurrent disease at the columella and right nasal ala (*B*). MMS was again used to remove the lesions, which resulted in a 9-mm columellar defect and a 5-mm right alar rim defect that were reconstructed with an FTSG from the left preauricular area. Scarring and telangiectasias were treated with combined pulsed dye laser and ablative Er:YAG fractional lasers with results seen 5 months after skin graft placement and 2 rounds of laser treatments (*C, D*) as well as 8 months postoperatively after 4 laser treatments (*E, F*). The patient chose not to undergo any additional intervention.

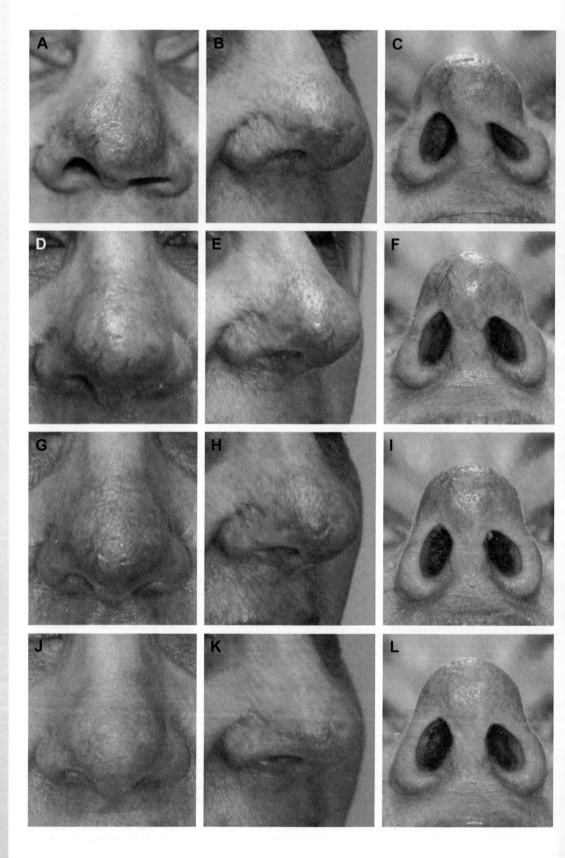

by more laser treatments to assist with tissue remodeling.

Laser fundamentals are beyond the scope of this article, but the advantage of laser therapy is that specific epidermal and dermal structures can be selectively targeted through precise selection of dosimetry, and as a noncontact technique there is no mechanical trauma to the skin.[8,10,11] In contrast, one limitation of dermabrasion (using sandpaper or rotary burrs) is that force is exerted on the tissue, and this may distract wounds. Hence, dermabrasion is seldom used during the acute phases of wound healing, and frequently it is used at 8 weeks.[10] Our laser treatment protocols begin on the day of suture removal, during the acute phase of wound healing.[8,9] We then select the appropriate wavelength and dosimetry parameters depending on what each injury requires and how it is likely to respond to treatment. A typical approach would start with pulsed dye laser therapy at suture removal with consideration of fractional ablative resurfacing 2 weeks later. Pulsed dye lasers target the scar vasculature. The fractional ablative resurfacing can be every 4 weeks for up to 5 treatments. At approximately 5 to 6 weeks, nonablative lasers maybe used at 2-week to 4-week intervals to support collagen remodeling.[8–10]

For early scar redness and erythema, a "vascular" laser, such as the 595-nm pulsed dye laser is used. Light from this laser is preferentially absorbed by hemoglobin.[8,9,12] Being nonablative, it creates no eschar for the patients to care for following treatment.[13] Scars will have many different-sized blood vessels and the laser settings can be adjusted to target each specifically. The pulse width can be set shorter for smaller vessels and longer for larger vessels. For general redness and erythema, we use settings similar to rosacea treatments: an energy density of 7.5 J/cm^2 with a 6-ms pulse width using a 10-mm spot size. We often make 2 passes to complete a single treatment. It is valuable to have a built-in cooling device or cooling technique to allow the epidermis to be cooled

selectively.[11] The laser we use is the V-Beam Perfecta (Syneron/Candela, Wayland, MA) with a 30/30 cooling setting (30 ms spurt of cryogen with a 30-ms delay until laser burst). For larger vessels and telangiectasias, the laser can be set to an energy density of 12.5 J/cm^2, 20-ms pulse width, and 30/30 cooling using a 7-mm spot size. Often a specific scar will get different treatment protocols at the same time depending on what is causing the erythema. It is important to allow the tissue to cool and to not be overly aggressive, as burns and blisters can occur.

For dermal collagen remodeling, the nonablative fractional 1550-nm wavelength lasers can be used[14] with multiple passes. This is often used in a fractional manner with multiple passes. Typically this laser is reserved for depressed scars that require multiple treatments to restore collagen over time. These lasers can generate significant temperature elevations, and without the traditional visual feedback of pinpoint bleeding seen with ablative lasers, burns and blisters are possible. It is important to wait at least 1 minute between each successive pass to allow the skin to thermally relax. A common setting used in our practice for nasal tip or dorsal scars is an energy of 45 mJ, treatment coverage area of 26% delivered with 6 passes. Again, it must be stressed to cool the superficial skin between each pass for extended periods (at least 1 minute with a cooling technique) to prevent burns and blistering.

Ablative lasers have the highest water absorption peaks and thus lead to destruction and removal of the superficial epidermal and dermal tissue.[8,9] In our practice, we use the 2940-nm wavelength Er:YAG laser with a tunable pulse duration. Er:YAG has high absorption in water, and thus a vertically shallow optical penetration depth. The 10,600-nm wavelength CO2 laser is also frequently used in this regard as well by many surgeons with excellent results, although thermal injury and depth of ablation are substantially deeper.[8,9,11] These ablative lasers are used in a fractional pattern of 11% to 22% treatment coverage area with multiple passes as desired.

Fig. 4. A 54-year-old woman with early rhinophyma presenting 5 years after Mohs excision of a right lateral nasal basal cell cancer with local reconstruction (performed elsewhere) and 3 years after subsequent rhinoplasty for persistent cosmetic defect (performed elsewhere). Note twisting of the tip and right alar rim notching from soft tissue triangle retraction (A), excessive columellar show (B), and nostril asymmetry with rightward deviation of the columella (C) and redness and telangiectasias in photographs at consultation. Her contour irregularities were treated with revision rhinoplasty with costal cartilage (septal extension graft, articulated alar rim grafts, lateral crural tensioning). Eight weeks postoperative enhanced telangiectasias of the nasal tip are seen (D–F). Telangiectasias were treated with a pulsed dye laser and the skin textural changes were treated with an ablative Erb:YAG fractional laser with results shown 3 weeks after the first treatment and 4 months postoperatively (G–I), as well as 11 weeks after the fourth treatment and 10 months postoperatively (J–L).

A standard protocol for a hypertrophic nasal scar is 500 μm of depth of ablation, 11% of fractional treatment coverage area delivered with 3 passes. Pinpoint bleeding will be obtained similar to dermabrasion. This protocol will require posttreatment wound care and prophylaxis at the discretion of the surgeon (**Fig. 2**).

Surgical Scar Revision

Surgical revision of nasal scars is indicated when the scar distorts the natural contours of the nose. A tight scar band can pull the ala medially for example. This can be released with a Z-plasty to reorient the scar and then followed by laser treatments as indicated to blend the incisions.

Depressed scars with resulting soft tissue defect can be replaced with a full-thickness skin graft (FTSG) to release the pull and straining created from contraction. **Fig. 3** shows an example of when an FTSG can be used to fill the soft tissue defect. Grafting can be followed by laser as stated previously to blend the areas. This patient elected to have no further treatment beyond the FTSG.

The soft tissue triangle area of the nose is a particular area of interest to the nasal surgeon. This web of tissue has the propensity to be easily distorted by scar. It is a classic scenario that the soft tissue triangle is scared leading to retraction and notching of the ala. This can be repaired with an auricular composite graft to supply the

needed rigid framework in conjunction with soft tissue simultaneously. Alar retraction is a common consequence of nasal reconstruction and trauma as well, and can be treated with composite grafts to the vestibular inner lining or by using structural rhinoplasty techniques, as seen in **Fig. 4**.

Injectable Steroids and Fillers

It is not our practice to use injectable fillers in the nose for scars, although many surgeons do report excellent results with such intervention. This topic is addressed in other sections of treating facial scars, as there are roles for such treatments in specific locations and instances.

Steroid injections are a commonly accepted method to settle inflammation and hypertrophy of scars. Our typical protocol is triamcinolone 40 mg/mL and volume is determined by the scar size. For 1 to 2 cm^2 = 20 to 40 mg/course, 2 to 6 cm^2 = 40 to 80 mg/course, 6 to 12 cm^2 = 80 to 120 mg/course. We inject at 1-week to 4-week intervals (2–3 injections total). The patient in **Fig. 5** demonstrates the utility of local steroid injections. As discussed within this article, most patients undergo a combination of treatments to maximize results.[15]

Total Subunit Reconstruction

Essentially after the previously discussed more conservative options have been considered or attempted, the final stage is total nasal subunit

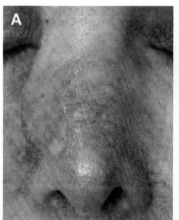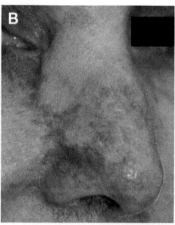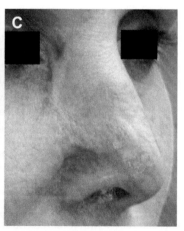

Fig. 5. A 52-year-old woman presents 3 months after excision of a right nasal sidewall basal cell carcinoma and reconstruction with a fascial-musculocutaneous glabellar (Banner) flap (performed elsewhere). One month after her surgery she noted thickening of the skin at the incision, was referred to the senior author (BJFW) for management, and underwent local injection of triamcinolone. (*A*) The patient at presentation after 1 treatment with injected triamcinolone. A second dose of triamcinolone (0.2 mL of Kenalog-40) was injected within the scar at this time. A third injection of triamcinolone was delivered 4 weeks later. (*B*) Two months after the third steroid injection and 1 month after her first session of laser skin resurfacing (by JSN). (*C*) Eleven months after initial reconstruction followed by 3 rounds of local steroid injections and multiple sessions of laser resurfacing.

reconstruction. If the scar is confined within one nasal subunit, often replacement of the entire subunit can lead to better results than having visible scars within the boundaries of a specific nasal subunit. Interpolated flaps such as a paramedian forehead or a melolabial flap are often used to replace the soft tissue when a significant volume is required. This is well established in the facial plastic surgery literature and is discussed with a patient example here. The patient in **Fig. 6** is a 53-year-old woman who underwent total nasal reconstruction after roughly 9 rhinoplasty operations (performed elsewhere).

PEARLS AND PITFALLS

Pearl: Let the tissue and scar define themselves before intervention.

Pitfall: Treating scars before allowing the tissue to demarcate will delay and distort the nasal structures and may mislead reconstructive efforts.

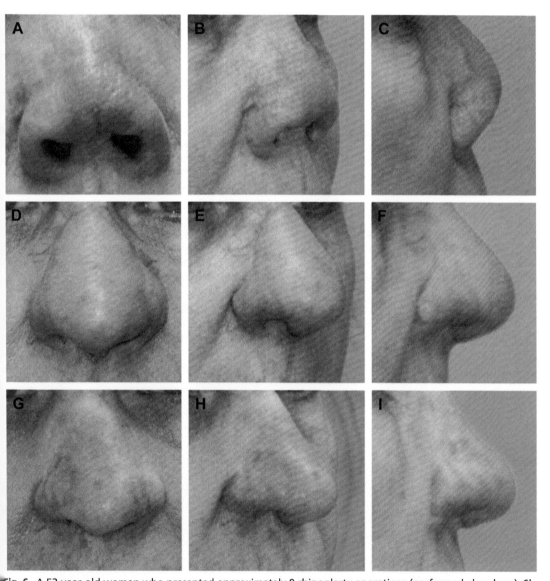

Fig. 6. A 53-year-old woman who presented approximately 9 rhinoplasty operations (performed elsewhere). She elected to undergo total nasal reconstruction with a paramedian forehead flap. Her procedure was performed in 3 stages with 5 minor additional refinement and defatting procedures performed under local.[16] Laser therapy was also provided. Images show presentation (*A–C*), 4 weeks after final staging of the paramedian forehead flap (*D–F*), and 4 years after final staging of paramedian forehead flap with 4 refinement procedures and 1 treatment of combination pulsed dye and fractional laser resurfacing (*G–I*).

Pearl: With laser energy, always be conservative. Slow and steady progress allows you to appreciate how the scar and the patient will respond to laser treatments.

Pitfall: Lasers are powerful devices. Being overly aggressive with the laser can worsen and create new scars.

REFERENCES

1. Dauwe PB, Pulikkottil BJ, Lavery L, et al. Does hyperbaric oxygen therapy work in facilitating acute wound healing: a systematic review. Plast Reconstr Surg 2014;133(2):208e–15e.

2. Manuskiatti W, Fitzpatrick RE. Treatment response of keloidal and hypertrophic sternotomy scars: comparison among intralesional corticosteroid, 5-fluorouracil, and 585-nm flashlamp-pumped pulsed-dye laser treatments. Arch Dermatol 2002; 138(9):1149–55.

3. Sidgewick GP, McGeorge D, Bayat A. A comprehensive evidence-based review on the role of topicals and dressings in the management of skin scarring. Arch Dermatol Res 2015; 307:461–77.

4. Shin TM, Bordeaux JS. The role of massage in scar management: a literature review. Dermatol Surg 2012;38:414–23.

5. Hultman CS, Friedstat JS, Edkins RE, et al. Laser resurfacing and remodeling of hypertrophic burn scars: the results of a large, prospective, before-after cohort study, with long-term follow-up. Ann Surg 2014;260(3):519–29.

6. Carniol PJ, Hamilton MM, Carniol ET. Current status of fractional laser resurfacing. JAMA Facial Plast Surg 2015;17(5):360–6.

7. El-Domyati M, Barakat M, Awad S, et al. Microneedling therapy for atrophic acne scars: an objective evaluation. J Clin Aesthet Dermatol 2015;8(7):36–42.

8. Oliaei S, Nelson JS, Fitzpatrick R, et al. Laser treatment of scars. Facial Plast Surg 2012;28(5):518–24.

9. Oliaei S, Nelson JS, Fitzpatrick R, et al. Use of lasers in acute management of surgical and traumatic incisions on the face. Facial Plast Surg Clin North Am 2011;19(3):543–50.

10. Leake DS, Baker SR. Scar revision and local flap refinement. In: Baker SR, editor. Local flaps in facial reconstruction. Philadelphia: Elsevier Inc; 2007. p. 727–66.

11. Wu EC, Wong BJF. Lasers and optical technology in facial plastic surgery. Arch Facial Plast Surg 2008; 10:381–409.

12. Cohen BE, Brauer JA, Geronemus RG. Acne scarring: a review of available therapeutic lasers. Lasers Surg Med 2016;48(2):95–115.

13. Finney R, Torbeck R, Saedi N. Non-ablative fractional resurfacing in the treatment of scar contracture. Lasers Surg Med 2016;48(2):170–3.

14. Friedmann DP, Tzu JE, Kauvar AN, et al. Treatment of facial photodamage and rhytides using a novel 1,565nm non-ablative fractional erbium-doped fiber laser. Lasers Surg Med 2016;48(2):174–80.

15. On HR, Lee SH, Lee YS, et al. Evaluating hypertrophic thyroidectomy scar outcomes after treatment with triamcinolone injections and copper bromide therapy. Lasers Surg Med 2015;47(6): 479–84.

16. Menick FJ. Aesthetic refinements in use of forehead for nasal reconstruction: the paramedian forehead flap. Clin Plast Surg 1990;17(4):607–22.

Treating Scars of the Chin and Perioral Region

Jessyka G. Lighthall, MD[a,b], Fred G. Fedok, MD[b,c,d],*

KEYWORDS

- Lip scar • Chin scar • Perioral scar • Scar revision • Reconstruction • Dermabrasion • Resurfacing
- Corticosteroid

KEY POINTS

- An understanding of the anatomy and function of the lips is critical for optimal scar revision and reconstructive results.
- Realistic expectations must be discussed with the patient preoperatively.
- Key anatomic landmarks should be meticulously realigned. Scars should be placed in borders of the aesthetic subunits and along resting skin tension lines.
- Resurfacing may be used to improve the appearance of irregular scars.
- Adjunctive therapies such as intralesional injection of corticosteroids or other agents, volume restoration, or botulinum toxin may be necessary to optimize results.

INTRODUCTION

Scars arise from a variety of etiologies in the perioral region. Although congenital causes exist, such as residual scarring after involution of a hemangioma, this is an uncommon cause of lower facial scarring. More commonly, treatment of congenital abnormalities such as cleft lip repair or treatment of vascular malformations causes scarring that may need to be revised. Much of the published literature focuses on improving the appearance of upper lip scarring in the cleft lip deformity population, including the need for secondary revision surgery to rectify lip length discrepancies, vermilion deficiencies, and irregularities of the vermilion border. Iatrogenic causes of scarring are also common in adults, primarily owing to resection of malignancy with reconstruction. Facial soft tissue trauma may result in adverse or irregular scarring of the lips or chin regions, with burns posing a particularly complex reconstructive dilemma. This article focuses on the treatment of scars in the lip and chin region.

PERTINENT ANATOMY

A thorough knowledge of facial anatomy, including that of the lip and chin, is critical for optimal aesthetic and functional outcomes. The perioral region includes the upper and lower lips as well as the chin. It is bordered laterally by the bilateral melolabial and labiomandibular creases and extends superiorly from the subnasale to the menton inferiorly. The perioral region encompasses the inferior one-third of the facial proportions and can be further subdivided with the upper lip accounting for one-third and the lower lip and chin accounting for two-thirds of the lower facial

Funding Source: None.
Conflicts of Interest: None.
[a] Division of Otolaryngology-Head & Neck Surgery, Penn State Hershey Medical Center, 500 University Drive H091, Hershey, PA 17033, USA; [b] Facial Plastic and Reconstructive Surgery, Penn State Hershey Medical Center, 500 University Drive H091, Hershey, PA 17033, USA; [c] Fedok Plastic Surgery, 113 East Fern Avenue, Foley, AL 36535, USA; [d] Department of Surgery, USA Medical Center, The University of South Alabama, 2451 Fillingim Street, Mobile, AL 36617, USA
* Corresponding author. Fedok Plastic Surgery, Facial Plastic and Reconstructive Surgery, 113 East Fern Avenue, Foley, AL 36535.
E-mail addresses: drfredfedok@me.com; drfedok@fedokplasticsurgery.com

facialplastic.theclinics.com

division[1,2] (**Fig. 1**). On profile, ideal lip projection is typically characterized as the upper lip extending 3.5 mm and the lower lip 2.2 mm anterior to a line between the subnasale and pogonion[3] (**Fig. 2**A) or the upper lip being 4 mm and lower lip 2 mm posterior to a line drawn between the nasal tip and pogonion (see **Fig. 2**B).[4] The ultimate position of the lips depends on the underlying skeletal and dental framework of the patient, aging and volume-related changes, and the muscular apparatus that suspends the lips and baseline skin characteristics.

The superficial perioral region incorporates the lip and chin aesthetic regions. The cutaneous lip aesthetic region is further subdivided into aesthetic units, including the paired upper lip lateral units, the philtrum, and the lower lip. The chin subunit extends superiorly from the mentolabial sulcus, the menton inferiorly, and the labiomandibular creases laterally.[5] Key features of the upper and lower lips include the vermilion, which is a modified mucosal lining making up the free margin of the lip.[6] The dry–wet border is the location at which the dry modified mucosal lining meets the wet mucosal lining of the lip. Where the white or cutaneous lip meets the red lip or vermilion is the vermilion border or white roll, which is a key anatomic landmark for reconstruction and scar revision of the lip (**Fig. 3**).

The lip lining incorporates the white or cutaneous lip and the vermilion externally with the labial mucosal as an internal lining. The bulk of the lip is made up of the orbicularis oris muscle, the fibers of which interconnect at the oral commissures at the modiolus, as well as subcutaneous tissue and minor salivary glands.[6] Other muscles of facial expression insert along the orbicularis or at the modiolus and assist with movement of the lips. The primary blood supply to the lips is from the superior and inferior labial arteries, branches of the facial arteries, which may be located posterior to the orbicularis muscle in a submucosal plane at approximately the level of the vermilion border with branches off these vessels also supplying the chin.[6] The superior and inferior labial arteries are useful for local axial flap reconstruction of the lips. The venous drainage is less well-defined and thought to parallel the arterial supply.

FUNCTIONAL ATTRIBUTES

In addition to the aesthetic implications and sensory function of the lips, there are multiple functional considerations with reconstruction. The mouth and lips are integral to production of facial expressions, provide oral competence during eating and drinking, are critical for proper articulation, and allow for specialized functions such as kissing.[6] Secondary reconstruction including management of scars should aim to restore oral competence and an innervated orbicularis sphincter to maintain proper lip function in addition to providing a cosmetically appealing result.

PATIENT EVALUATION

Before undergoing any procedure for scar revision, a complete history and head and neck physical examination should be performed to assess the appropriateness of the patient for a procedure, including the etiology of the scar condition. Comorbidities, including poorly controlled diabetes, immunosuppression, autoimmune or inflammatory disorder, tobacco abuse, history of radiation therapy, status of treatment of existing malignancies, history of keloid or hypertrophic scarring, and history of cold sores, should be identified and considered during treatment planning. A history of prior procedures to improve scar appearance should be acquired. Patient desires should be elucidated and establishment of realistic expectations is paramount before proceeding with intervention.

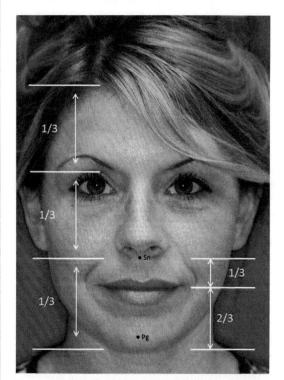

Fig. 1. Vertical dimensions of the face. The inferior one-third is divided into the upper lip (one-third) and the lower lip and chin (two-thirds). Pg, pogonion; Sn, subnasale.

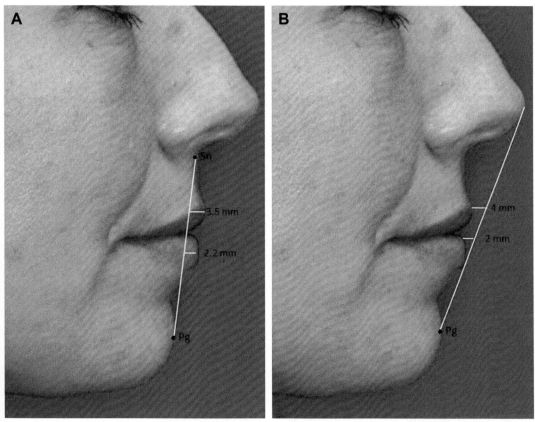

Fig. 2. Ideal horizontal lip projection. (*A*) Projection measured relative to line extending from subnasale to pogonion. (*B*) Lip position measured relative to line between nasal tip and pogonion. Pg, pogonion; Sn, subnasale.

SUBUNIT ORGANIZED APPROACH TO SCAR AND DEFORMITY MANAGEMENT

Secondary reconstruction should attempt to maintain all aesthetic, sensory, and motor functions of the lip, similar to primary reconstruction of perioral defects. Scarring of the lip may be minor and treated with small superficial revisions and adjunctive procedures, or include large secondary deformities with volume discrepancy requiring a more extensive reconstruction. In severely contracted scars of the lip with volume deficiency, this may be the optimal option for function and appearance. Full-thickness resection and revision should be performed when necessary and revision may follow published algorithms for defect reconstruction.[6,7] Briefly, full-thickness defects involving less than 30% the width of the upper or lower lip are considered small and are amenable to primary closure.[8,9] Defects 30% to 60% the width of the lip are intermediate sized defects and in general require a pedicled cross-lip flap as primary closure will result in microstomia. Finally, large defects greater than 60% lip width will require adjacent flaps from the cheek or free tissue transfer.[8,9] When full-thickness reconstruction is performed, reestablishing the orbicularis sphincter is critical if at all possible to maintain adequate function.

Similar to other regions of the face, when planning reconstruction or scar revision of the perioral region, it is important to place incisions parallel to relaxed skin tension lines (RSTLs) if possible. In the

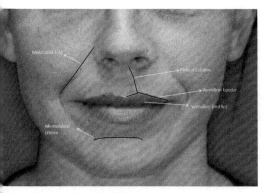

Fig. 3. Key landmarks of the perioral region.

lips, these are radially distributed perpendicular to the orbicularis oris muscle action.[6] Patient age should be taken into account; with aging comes the appearance of static vertical lip lines, muscle atrophy, loss of defining points, and loss of lip volume and lip definition.[2] Therefore, the appearance of scars and need for revision will vary based on age. Whenever possible, scars should be placed along aesthetic unit borders and reconstruction may require excision of remaining uninvolved tissue of an aesthetic subunit to maximize scar camouflage. Finally, meticulous alignment of the vermilion border is critical for minimizing the appearance of scars. An organized approach to scar and deformity management based on a subunit approach will be discussed.

Upper White Lip

Scars of the cutaneous (white) white lip are more apparent when they cross aesthetic units, cause a trap door deformity, exhibit contracture with volume and lip height discrepancies, distort key landmarks (eg, philtrum), are depressed or elevated, are widened, do not have a complete orbicularis sphincter, or are alopecic in males. Many different treatments exist and often a combination of surgical and adjunctive maneuvers is necessary to provide an optimal aesthetic and functional result. Scars with irregular height or thickness compared with the surrounding tissue may be improved with resurfacing techniques alone such as laser therapy or mechanical dermabrasion (discussed elsewhere in this paper).[10] Widened but appropriately oriented scars in RSTLs may be treated with a fusiform excision and revised with meticulous soft tissue handling techniques.[11] If possible, a simple elliptical excision may be performed. For upper lip scars with a large widened area, excision may involve resection of normal surrounding skin, including the entire aesthetic subunit when necessary. Closure should attempt to place the new

incision line within the borders of aesthetic subunits, for example, around the alar base or within the melolabial fold (**Fig. 4** provides an example of incision placement for subunit replacement). Larger resections may require adjacent transposition flaps or advancement of surrounding tissue for cutaneous closure.[6,7] For total upper lip scarring secondary to burns or caustic injuries, cutaneous excision of the entire cutaneous lip aesthetic region with reconstruction by a full-thickness skin graft may be required.[12]

Scars crossing the RSTLs or with minor stepoffs at the vermilion border will benefit from revision using a Z-plasty technique (discussed elsewhere in this paper) to lengthen, reorient, and irregularize the scar.[13] Asking a patient to purse her or his lips will allow for assessment of the status of the underlying orbicularis oris muscle sphincter. Inadequate realignment of the muscle during initial reconstruction may lead to a depressed scar, notching of the lip, or a scar that is more visible with dynamic lip function. In such cases, it is necessary not only revise the scar, but to also address the underlying orbicularis muscle. For upper lip scars that exhibit significant vertical height discrepancies, as may be the case after primary cleft lip repair, complete lip revision and reconstruction with a rotation–advancement technique may be necessary.

Scars with significant contraction involving all layers, severe whistle deformities, as an adjunct in secondary cleft lip revisions, or for a tight lip with limited mobility affecting function, full-thickness wedge resection with layered closure or local flap reconstruction may be appropriate. If necessary, a W- or M-plasty is designed with the wedge resection to avoid crossing aesthetic boundaries.[6]

Intermediate-sized defects of the upper lip pose a unique challenge to reconstruct without causing microstomia. If less than one-half of the width of the upper lip, full-thickness bilateral lip

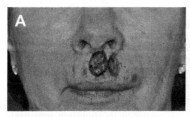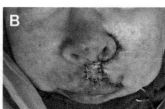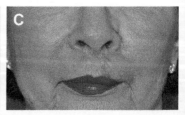

Fig. 4. Clinical and intraoperative images depicting the use of several techniques to limit unfavorable scarring and deformity after excision of cancer from the upper lip. (*A*) Clinical image depicting patient's resultant defect after excision of 2 small malignancies of the upper lip. (*B*) Intraoperative image of patient after incision and advancement of left upper lip tissues at vermilion border, crescentic excision of left perialar cheek tissue to allow medial advancement of left upper lip tissues and full-thickness skin graft of defect of the philtrum. (*C*) Clinical image depicting patient 8 weeks after repair.

advancements may be performed and will require perialar crescentric excisions to allow adequate lateral lip segment mobilization.[6] For defects of the upper lip involving 30% to 60% of the width that do not involve the oral commissure, a full-thickness cross-lip pedicled flap (Abbe lip-switch flap) may be used (**Fig. 5**).[6,8,9,12,14] The Abbe or extended Abbe flap is pedicled on the labial artery and designed to fill the unique shape of the defect, with a 1:1 match of defect height but typically 50% of the width to minimize upper and lower lip width discrepancy. The flap is rotated 180° and inset in layers with layered closure of the donor site. After adequate time for vascularization, a second stage procedure to divide the pedicle is performed. Often, this type of flap is combined with additional treatments to provide optimal aesthetic results for scar revision (**Fig. 6**). For intermediate defects involving the oral commissure, the Estlander cross-lip flap is useful (**Fig. 7**).[6,7] This flap is also based on the labial artery and allows for a 1-stage pedicled reconstruction of the lateral lip and commissure. However, it does lead to blunting of the oral commissure with fullness, which may require secondary revision. For near-total or total upper lip defects, more unique flaps should be considered, such as bilateral McGregor or Gilles fan flaps that use adjacent cheek tissue for reconstruction, staged melolabial flaps, pedicled temporoparietal scalp flap, or free tissue transfer.[6]

The Chin and Lower Lip

In the lower lip and chin regions, incisions should be placed at the labiomandibular lines and at the labiomental crease. Similar concepts to scar revision and defect management in the upper lip exist for the lower lip. Wedge resections with or without W-plasties are appropriate for excision of scarring or contracture involving less than one-third of the lower lip.[15] For defects up to 50% of the width, bilateral lower lip full-thickness advancement may be performed with good results with the inferior incision designed in the mental crease.[6,9] As discussed, Abbe or Estlander cross-lip flaps may be similarly used to reconstruct lower lip defects of 30% to 60% of the lower lip.[6,8,9,15] These and defects may also be repaired by one of many flap techniques using tissues from surrounding cheek and lip skin. Partial thickness circumoral rotation–advancement (Karapandzic) flaps that preserve the neurovascular bundles during dissection of facial muscular attachments off the orbicularis oris muscle are a useful technique to reconstruct large defects of the lower lip, and less commonly the upper lip (**Fig. 8**).[16] This provides an innervated reconstruction that attempts to reestablish the oribicularis sphincter and provide oral competence.[6,9] The Gilles fan flap and the McGregor modification of the Gilles flap are full-thickness flaps with incisions beginning at the inferior aspect of the defect and narrowly pedicled on the ipsilateral oral commissure to provide a composite lip rotation–advancement flap with a layered closure (**Fig. 9**).[6,9] Bilateral flaps may be used to reconstruct large defects and restores the orbicularis muscle sphincter. Blunting of the oral commissure and microstomia will result.

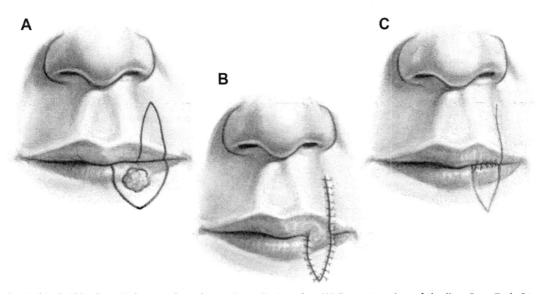

Fig. 5. (*A–C*) Abbe lip switch procedure. (*From* Cupp CL, Larrabee W. Reconstruction of the lips. Oper Tech Otolaryngol Head Neck Surg 1993;4(1):46–53; with permission.)

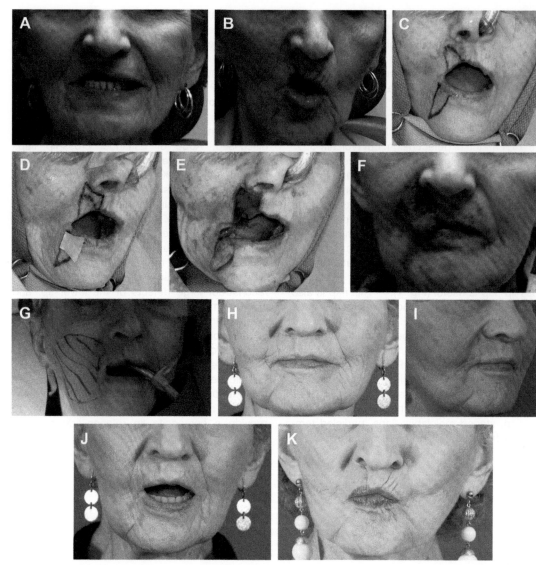

Fig. 6. Use of multiple reconstructive techniques to improve the form and function of a patients right upper lip after a previous cancer operation. (*A, B*) Clinical images of patient presenting with atrophy of right upper lip occurring after limited maxillectomy on the right. On examination, the patient's lip was focally dennervated with a loss of muscle mass, vertical contracture, and with impairment of oral competence. (*C*) Intraoperative image of initial surgical plan for an Abbe lip switch procedure to replace atrophied and contracted region of right upper lip with bulkier tissue from the lower lip. (*D, E*) Intraoperative image of patient depicting final surgical plan for lip switch using template transfer of upper lip subunit to lower lip. (Note: the foil template is positioned to reflect rotation and inversion of proposed lip segment) The majority of upper lip lining was preserved to aid in the retention upper lip length. Note the placement of incisions in the labiomandibular crease and adjacent to the philtral column. (*F*) Clinical image depicting the patient at an intermediate stage of reconstruction before the lip pedicle was divided. (*G*) Intraoperative image of patient, several weeks after pedicle division, depicting surgical planning for fat transfer to restore loss of volume of lower cheek and white lip, flap inset was also revised at the time. (*H–K*) Clinical images depicting the patient and final result of the multiple interventions.

For large lower lip defects, Bernard von Burow flaps may be designed, which use bilateral cheek advancement flaps, requiring excision of Burow's triangles adjacent to the oral commissures to allow full-thickness cheek advancement (**Fig. 10**).[6] This technique and variations thereof also requires mucosal advancement over the free edge to reconstruct the vermilion and does not reconstruct the oral sphincter. Finally, total lower lip reconstruction typically requires at a minimum a regional

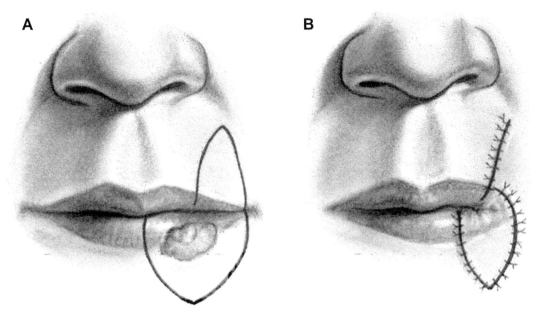

Fig. 7. (*A, B*) Estlander flap. (*From* Cupp CL, Larrabee W. Reconstruction of the lips. Oper Tech Otolaryngol Head Neck Surg 1993;4(1):46–53; with permission.)

flap such as the submental island flap[17,18] or free tissue transfer.[19,20]

The Vermilion or Red Lip

Isolated scar contraction, notching, or volume deficiency of the vermilion may be treated with direct excision, local tissue rearrangement, free autografts, alloplasts, xenografts, or any combination of these approaches.[21] Although most published research focuses on secondary deformities owing to repair of cleft lip defects, the tenants hold true for vermilion deficiencies owing to any etiology of scarring and may be responsible for a persistently poor aesthetic outcome of an

otherwise excellent lip repair. Deficiencies without a significant component of pars marginalis deficiency may be repaired by Z-plasty, V–Y labial mucosal advancement flaps, or mucosal transposition flaps may be useful.[6,10,13,22,23] A Z-plasty may be useful in the vermilion to add bulk or to realign the wet–dry border.[13] A single or multiple V–Y advancements may be used to improve the aesthetic appearance of the red lip and provide bulk owing to scar contracture. This flap involves creating a V-shaped incision extending from the apex of the scar or volume deficiency that extends along the labial mucosa.[6,22,24] It is then advanced into the deficiency with primary closure of the donor site, resulting in an overall Y-shaped

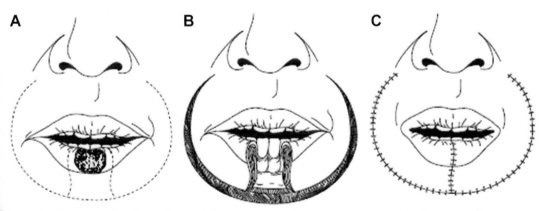

Fig. 8. (*A–C*) Karapandzic flaps. (*From* Ishii LE, Byrne PJ. Lip reconstruction. Facial Plast Surg Clin North Am 2009;17(3):445–53; with permission.)

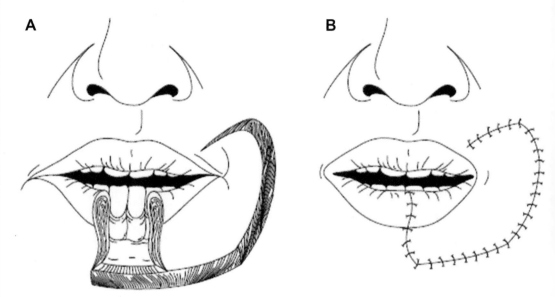

Fig. 9. (*A, B*) Gilles fan flap. (*From* Ishii LE, Byrne PJ. Lip reconstruction. Facial Plast Surg Clin North Am 2009;17(3):445–53; with permission.)

appearance of the incision line. Although less common, if excess unilateral bulk exists, direct elliptical excision may be useful to improve symmetry. For deficiencies of the vermilion, including malposition, a mucosal advancement flap may be warranted and is often used in conjunction with other procedures (**Figs. 11** and **12**).

When a significant amount of vermilion bulk is needed, a laterally based full-thickness vermilion advancement flap that includes the pars marginalis of the orbicularis oris muscle may also be used and is a 1-stage procedure.[6] It does, however, require a lengthy incision along the vermilion border and risks visible scarring in the region.

Additionally, multiple pedicled flaps for vermilion reconstruction have been described, including vermilion cross-lip pedicled flaps,[6,25,26] mutual cross-lip musculomucosal flaps,[27] facial artery myomucosal flaps,[28] or ventral tongue flaps.[29] These procedures require a second stage for division and inset of the pedicle and do carry a risk of secondary volume deficiency of the donor site or poor color mismatch of the donor and recipient tissue.

Finally, for severe vermilion volume deficiencies secondary to scar contraction or inadequate muscle approximation, a complete revision of a previously repaired cleft lip may be indicated or a

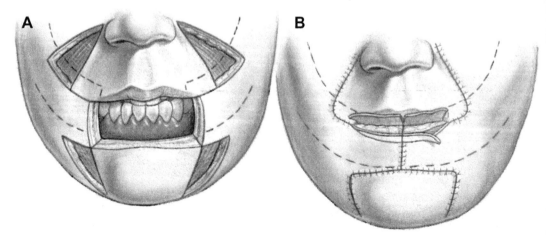

Fig. 10. (*A, B*) Webster modification of the Bernard von Burow flap. (*From* Cupp CL, Larrabee W. Reconstruction of the lips. Oper Tech Otolaryngol Head Neck Surg 1993;4(1):46–53; with permission.)

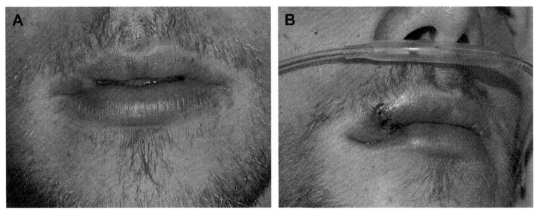

Fig. 11. The use of Z-plasty and tissue advancement to improve the appearance of lip scar. (*A*) Preoperative clinical image depicting the patient with a lip scar involving the malalignment of the orbicularis muscle, the vermilion and the vermilion border. (*B*) Intraoperative image of patient after Z-plasty to realign the vermilion border and the undermining and advancement of the red lip.

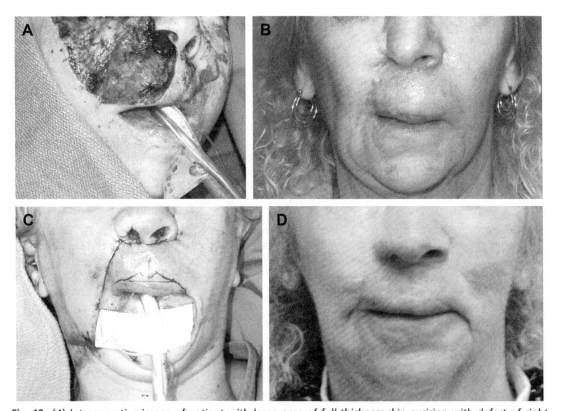

Fig. 12. (*A*) Intraoperative image of patient with large area of full-thickness skin excision with defect of right cheek, right nasal sidewall, and right upper lip. The right upper lip defect includes portions of the red lip, orbicularis oris muscle, cupids bow, and philtral column. (*B*) Clinical image depicting patient after extensive first-stage reconstruction. The lip has several asymmetries, including displacement of the cupids bow and scar contractures. (*C*) Intraoperative image of patient after scar revision and advancement of subnasale and right melolabial fold. The patients lip is marked for red lip advancement for creation of the cupids bow. (*D*) Clinical image of patient depicting results of scar revision and lip advancement.

full-thickness wedge resection of a severely scarred with muscle repair may be the best option to reconstruct the orbicularis sling with meticulous approximation of the vermilion border and dry–wet junction. Although typically well-tolerated, large wedge resections will cause microstomia and patients who wear dentures may be unable to do so after surgery.

The Vermilion Border

Discrepancies secondary to scarring along the vermilion border may be minor and range from a small stepoff to a large discrepancy of lip height requiring full-thickness revision. For minor discrepancies, direct elliptical or diamond-shaped scar excision with undermining and meticulous realignment of the vermilion border may be appropriate. For small stepoffs, a Z-plasty may be appropriate to realign the scar at the vermilion border (see **Fig. 11**).

The Oral Commissure

Scarring, blunting, and contractures of the oral commissure are difficult to treat, particularly with burn or caustic injuries, for which treatment may include splinting to minimize the need for future commissuroplasty.[30] For a blunted or scarred commissure after surgical defect reconstruction, a simple technique involves making a full-thickness horizontal incision at the level of the commissure or excising the scar to the desired location of the reconstructed commissure. The skin superior and inferior to the incision is then deepithelialization and mucosal advancement flaps are then used to reconstruct the vermilion.[6,9,31] A vermillion transposition flap technique may also be used.[32] In this technique, a triangular skin excision lateral to the commissure is performed with development of an upper or lower lip vermillion transposition flap that pivots into the defect to create the point of the commissure. A mucosal advancement flap is then created to fill the donor site defect and complete the commissuroplasty. For a more advanced procedure, the scar at the oral commissure is excised and buccal mucosal flaps are used either as a rotation–advancement flap or as a posteriorly based pedicled flap to recreate the commissure.[31,33] Finally, when a significant amount of tissue or bulk is necessary, an anteriorly based ventral tongue flap may be performed to recreate the commissure.[31,34] This procedure requires a second stage for division and inset of the flap and the color match tends to be poor, so it is typically reserved for more complex cases.

SPECIFIC TECHNIQUES
Z-plasty

A Z-plasty, or double transposition flap, is a useful technique to reorient a scar to better align with RSTLs or with a subunit border, improve the appearance of the vermilion border, irregularize an obvious scar for camouflage, lengthen the scar, or decrease contracture or webbing oftissues.[13,35] A classic simple Z-plasty is designed with the central limb consisting of the existing scar to be excised. At each end of the fusiform excision is a peripheral limb of equal length, running parallel to each other, with each limb ideally designed less than 1 cm in length for maximal scar camouflage (**Fig. 13**).[11,35] The angle between the central and peripheral limbs will vary based on the degree of reorientation and lengthening of the scar (**Table 1**). The incisions are created and triangular flaps undermined, transposed, and closed in layers. For longer scars, contracted scars, or curvilinear pincushion scars, multiple Z-plasties or "running" Z-plasties may be designed to disperse tension across the wound and provide irregularization for improved camouflage.[11]

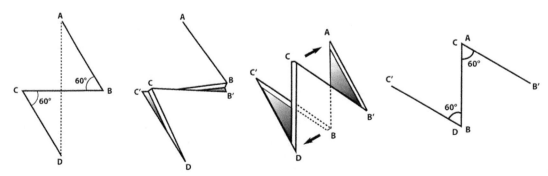

Fig. 13. The 60° Z-plasty transposition flaps. (*From* Shockley WW. Scar revision techniques: z-plasty, w-plasty, and geometric broken line closure. Facial Plast Surg Clin North Am 2011;19(3):455–63; with permission.)

Table 1
Standard angles between central and peripheral limbs of Z-plasty with corresponding percent lengthening of scar

Angle	Percent Lengthening
30°	25
45°	50
60°	75

In the perioral region, Z-plasties are frequently used to improve alignment of the vermilion border, break up a vertical scar, minimize contracture on surrounding tissues such as the alar base, and treat webbing around the oral commissure. In such circumstances or when attempting to align borders with different lip heights, it may be necessary to design Z-plasties with differential limb lengths or angles to effect the desired adjustments.[13]

W-plasty

W-plasty is a form of scar revision intended to create a regularly irregularized and reoriented scar for improved camouflage without lengthening the original scar (**Fig. 14**).[11] It is designed with a series of triangular flaps with short limbs surrounding the original scar and involves excision of additional uninvolved tissue. Undermining of the flaps is undertaken then the bilateral triangular flaps are advanced and interdigitated. W-plasty works well for shorter scars in the chin region, but is less well-suited for revision of lip scars or long scars as the regular pattern may result in the scar still being noticeable.[35]

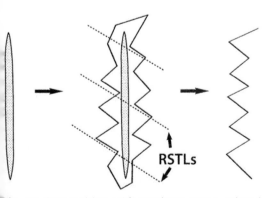

Fig. 14. Scar revision with W-plasty. RSTLs, relaxed skin tension lines. (*From* Shockley WW. Scar revision techniques: z-plasty, w-plasty, and geometric broken line closure. Facial Plast Surg Clin North Am 2011;19(3):455–63; with permission.)

Geometric Broken Line Closure

The geometric broken line closure allows for the reorientation of scars into the RSTLs but also provides an irregularly irregular resulting scar (**Fig. 15**). It involves excision of uninvolved tissue surrounding the scar, but incorporates a random pattern of small geometric shapes as advancement flaps. With the random pattern, the resulting scar becomes less noticeable and this pattern is therefore ideally suited to longer scars in an area with additional skin laxity to allow for additional skin excision.[35]

ADJUNCTS TO SCAR REVISION
Dermabrasion

Several methods exist to provide improve contour irregularities of scars. Dermabrasion is a mechanical resurfacing technique typically performed with a diamond fraise aligned perpendicular to the scar and provide gentle feathering of surrounding tissue.[36] Alternatively, dermabrasion may be performed with a wire brush or manually with dermasanding. All these techniques involve removing the epidermis and a portion of the papillary dermis grossly visualized as pinpoint bleeding.[10,36] The superficial reticular dermis is reached when a yellowish-white color is encountered. Subsequent reepithelialization is driven by adnexal structures and surrounding epithelium to provider a smoother appearance of scars with contour irregularities or excess thickness. Abrading into the reticular dermis may lead to adverse scarring because injury to adnexal structures key for reepithelialization may occur.[36] Other potential complications include prolonged erythema or pigmentary changes.

Laser

Lasers are commonly used to improve the appearance of perioral scars. A nice review of the utility of different types of lasers for treatment of scar was published by Sobanko and Alster in 2011.[37] The type of laser used and specific settings for scar revision depends on the individual scar characteristics. In general, laser therapy provides thermal wounding of the target tissue, which promotes subsequent neocollagenesis and collagen remodeling to provide the desired effect. Although spot treatment of the individual scar may be used, there is some benefit to treating the entire perioral aesthetic region for overall improved appearance. Briefly, for hypertrophic or keloid scars, treatment with the vascular-specific 525-nm pulse dye laser is most beneficial.[37] For other facial scars, including atrophic scars, ablative or nonablative

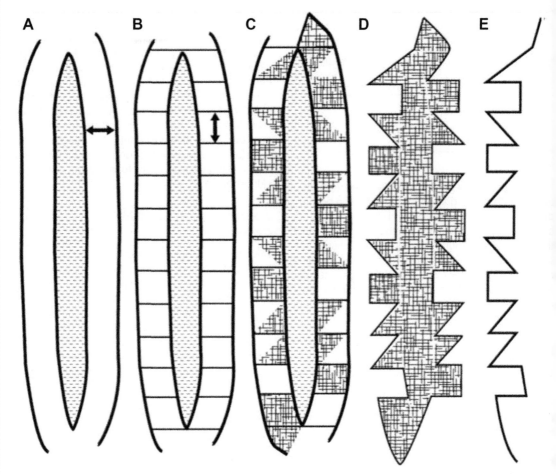

Fig. 15. (*A–E*) Scar revision with geometric broken line closure. (*From* Shockley WW. Scar revision techniques: z-plasty, w-plasty, and geometric broken line closure. Facial Plast Surg Clin North Am 2011;19(3):455–63; with permission.)

fractional laser therapy may be used with good results, with the type of laser system and settings varying based on scar and patient characteristics to maximize results and minimize the risk of adverse effects and downtime.[37] Laser therapy is commonly used as an adjunct to scar revision (**Figs. 16** and **17**).

Volume Restoration with Grafts or Filler

For vermilion volume deficiencies that persist despite techniques noted previously, or to resolve small remaining volume defects, some authors have reported using volumizing grafts alone or in conjunction with local flaps for treating persistent vermilion deficiencies. Many free autologous grafts have been discussed in the literature for both cosmetic and reconstructive purposes, including fat,[38,39] temporalis or temporoparietal fascia,[21,40,41] vermilion,[42] labia minora,[43] superficial musculoaponeurotic system,[40] sternocleidomastoid muscle and fascia,[44]

galea,[45] free composite myomucosal tongue,[46] and deepithelialized dermal grafts (**Fig. 18**). Proponents of these grafts note long-lasting and natural appearing results. Other grafts that have been used as adjuncts include acellular dermal matrix,[38,47] expanded polytetrafluoroethylene,[48] and a variety of temporary and permanent injectable materials to aid in volume augmentation when necessary.[49] Ideally, the use of a material requiring little morbidity for placement, providing long-lasting results and with minimal complications is ideal.

Botulinum Toxin

Botulinum toxin A is frequently used chemodenervation agent for the temporary treatment of dynamic facial rhytids. In recent years, its potential role in improving facial scars has been evaluated.[50–53] Because scars may widen or become hypertrophic when undue tension across a wound is applied during the healing process, it has been

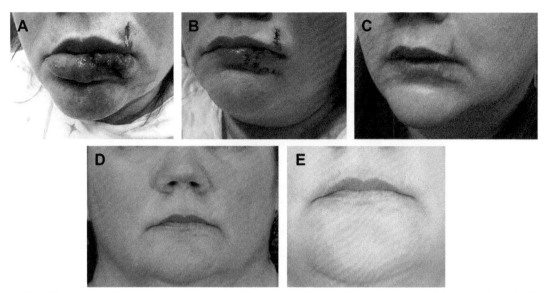

Fig. 16. Clinical and intraoperative images depicting the use of several techniques to provide optimal care in the prevention and management of perioral scarring after trauma. (*A*) Preoperative clinical image depicting the patient with a complicated lip laceration involving the orbicularis muscle and vermillion border. (*B*) Intraoperative image of patient after initial conservative debridement and 3-layer closure with precision alignment of vermilion border. (*C*) Clinical image depicting the patient 1 month after the procedure depicting hypertrophic scars. (*D, E*) Clinical image depicting the patient 1 year after the initial injury depicting result after the sequential use of pulsed dye laser and fractional CO_2 resurfacing.

postulated that temporary paralysis of muscles aligned perpendicular to wounds may decrease tension produced by muscle contraction.[52] Animal and human studies have suggested that placement of botulinum toxin at the time of scar revision improves the appearance of facial scars, including several prospective, blinded studies comparing results with a control group who received placebo.[50–52,54,55] A recent metaanalysis of randomized controlled trials of botulinum toxin A to treat hypertrophic scars (9 studies) found that it was significant in reducing the width of scars, improving patient satisfaction, and improvement

of scars on visual analog scales.[53] The authors do caution that, based on the heterogeneity of the patient population, the limited number of studies available for inclusion, and the potential for bias within the studies evaluated, additional high-quality research is necessary to further elucidate the role botulinum toxin A has in the prevention and treatment of adverse scars.

Intralesional Injections

Intralesional dermal injections are typically reserved for the treatment of aberrant scarring causing keloids or hypertrophic scars. Serial

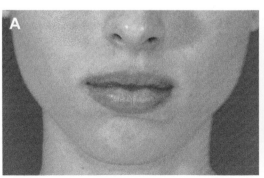
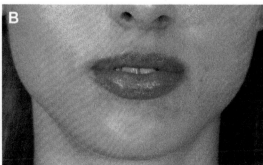

Fig. 17. Clinical image depicting of patient with mature scar of lower lip area that is depressed, erythematous, and irregular. (*A*) Preoperative photo. (*B*) Patient after scar excision and revision, fat transfer, and fractional laser resurfacing.

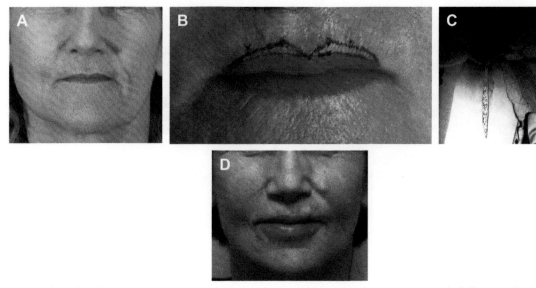

Fig. 18. Clinical and intraoperative images depicting the use of several techniques to provide fullness to the lip and to change the vermillion border. (Note: This is an elective case and not one owing to scarring, but the same techniques are used to improve the form of the lip in nonelective situations.) (*A*) Preoperative clinical image depicting the patient with a thin upper lip. (*B*) Intraoperative image of patient with surgical markings for incision and advancement of vermillion border. (Note: The incision is made just outside the natural vermilion border to preserve the fine detail.) (*C*) Intraoperative image of patient depicting the removal of a scar from a previous abdominal procedure. The excised scar graft will be deepithelized to be used as graft material and then tunneled through the upper lip to provide bulk. (*D*) Clinical image depicting the patient 1 month after the procedure.

intralesional corticosteroid injections, primarily with triamcinolone, have been used to treat hypertrophic scars and keloids with good results and remain a mainstay of treatment but may cause dermal atrophy, pigmentary changes, or striae.[10] Intralesional fluorouracil, an antimetabolite medication, has also shown good results in treating these scar groups alone or in combination with other therapies and is typically well-tolerated with a low side effect profile.[10]

Another agent deserving mention but in need of additional research evaluating its benefit in the treatment of hypertrophic scars and keloids is bleomycin. Bleomycin is a cytotoxic antibiotic that binds to DNA and induces strand breakage, although its specific mechanism in scar reduction is unknown. Although limited, existing literature suggests a potential role in improving the appearance of hypertrophic scars and decreasing recurrence of keloids.[10] In general, additional high-quality research is needed to help clarify the role of injectable agents in scar treatment.

Topical Agents

Commonly used agents discussed in the literature, including vitamin E or gels of onion extract have shown little to no improvement of scar cosmesis when compared with petroleum ointment alone.[56] Topical imiquimod cream, an immunomodulatory drug, has shown some limited improvement in scar appearance; however local side effects and occasional systemic effects of flu like symptoms have limited its widespread use and additional research is necessary to evaluate its role in the treatment of scars.[56]

Silicone gel sheeting

Silicone gel sheeting is often used in the prevention and treatment of hypertrophic scars and keloids. The exact mechanism of action is unknown, although common theories include provision of an occlusive and hydrated environment or improvement in oxygen tension.[56] Although multiple studies have performed literature reviews and recommend silicone gel sheeting in the treatment of hypertrophic or keloid scars to improve color, texture, and thickness,[56,57] a 2013 Cochrane review noted that available research is of poor quality and prone to bias, thus restricting the ability to make definitive conclusions regarding the effectiveness of silicone gel sheeting.[58]

Camouflage

For scarring around the lips and chin in males, scar camouflaging with hair transplantation is a useful adjunctive procedure to minimize the appearance of scars. Both single-hair transplantation and follicular unit grafting have been shown to improve the appearance of cleft lip and perioral scars.[59,60] For female patients, cosmetics can significantly assist in camouflaging of scars. Consideration should also be given to micropigmentation, or tattooing, to improve the camouflaging of perioral scars and mucocutaneous lip reconstruction, provide a more consistent vermilion border, and decrease the appearance of alopecia in appropriately selected patients.[61]

SUMMARY

Meticulous tissue handling techniques, proper alignment of scars whenever possible, and a tension-free closure and key in preventing adverse scarring. Before scar revision, realistic expectations should be firmly set with patients and overall goals discussed. Surgical revision is necessary for keloid scars not responding to conservative therapy, to reorient a scar into the RSTLs or place into the border of an aesthetic subunit, to decrease the width of scars, to irregularize a scar, or to correct volume discrepancies and contractures. Resurfacing is useful to improve contour irregularities and blend the scar with surrounding skin. Multiple adjunctive therapies are available and scar treatment should be individualized based on patient and scar characteristics. Often multimodality and serial therapy is necessary to optimize scar appearance.

REFERENCES

1. Ridley M, VanHook SM. Aesthetic facial proportions. In: Papel ID, editor. Facial plastic and reconstructive surgery. 3rd edition. New York: Thieme; 2009. p. 119–33.
2. Perkins SW, Sandel HD 4th. Anatomic considerations, analysis, and the aging process of the perioral region. Facial Plast Surg Clin North Am 2007; 15(4):403–7, v.
3. Burstone CJ. Lip posture and its significance in treatment planning. Am J Orthod 1967;53(4):262–84.
4. Powell N, Humphreys B. Proportions of the aesthetic face. New York: Thieme-Stratton; 1984.
5. Baker SR, editor. Local flaps in facial reconstruction. 2nd edition. Philadelphia: Mosby; 2007. p. 71–105.
6. Renner GJ. Reconstruction of the lip. In: Baker S, editor. Local flaps in facial reconstruction. 2nd edition. Philadelphia: Mosby; 2007. p. 475–524.
7. DeFatta RJ, Williams EF III. Lip reconstruction. In: Papel ID, editor. Facial plastic and reconstructive surgery. Third edition. New York: Thieme; 2009. p. 841–54.
8. Ishii LE, Byrne PJ. Lip reconstruction. Facial Plast Surg Clin North Am 2009;17(3):445–53.
9. Matin MB, Dillon J. Lip reconstruction. Oral Maxillofac Surg Clin North Am 2014;26(3):335–57.
10. Thomas JR, Somenek M. Scar revision review. Arch Facial Plast Surg 2012;14(3):162–74.
11. Kokoska M, Thomas JR. Scar revision. In: Papel ID, editor. Facial plastic and reconstructive surgery. 3rd edition. New York: Thieme; 2009. p. 59–65.
12. Weerda H. Reconstructive facial plastic surgery: a problem-solving manual. 1st edition. New York: Thieme; 2001.
13. Wentzell JM, Lund JJ. Z-plasty innovations in vertical lip reconstructions. Dermatol Surg 2011;37(11): 1646–62.
14. Kriet JD, Cupp CL, Sherris DA, et al. The extended abbe flap. Laryngoscope 1995;105(9 Pt 1):988–92.
15. McCarn KE, Park SS. Lip reconstruction. Otolaryngol Clin North Am 2007;40(2):361–80.
16. Karapandzic M. Reconstruction of lip defects by local arterial flaps. Br J Plast Surg 1974;27(1):93–7.
17. Guo Y, Mao C. The use of submental island flap for total lower lip reconstruction: a case report. Facial Plast Surg 2016;32(2):238–9.
18. Kim JP, Park HW, Park JJ, et al. Reconstruction after resection of a lower lip squamous cell carcinoma with a submental island flap. Ear Nose Throat J 2015;94(12):E19–21.
19. Bai S, Li RW, Xu ZF, et al. Total and near-total lower lip reconstruction: 20 years experience. J Craniomaxillofac Surg 2015;43(3):367–72.
20. Silberstein E, Krieger Y, Shoham Y, et al. Total lip reconstruction with tendinofasciocutaneous radial forearm flap. ScientificWorldJournal 2014;2014:219728.
21. Chen PK, Noordhoff MS, Chen YR, et al. Augmentation of the free border of the lip in cleft lip patients using temporoparietal fascia. Plast Reconstr Surg 1995;95(5):781–8 [discussion: 789].
22. Robinson DW, Ketchum LD, Masters FW. Double V-Y procedure for whistling deformity in repaired cleft lips. Plast Reconstr Surg 1970;46(3):241–4.
23. Matsuo K, Fujiwara T, Hayashi R, et al. Bilateral lateral vermilion border transposition flaps to correct the "whistling lip" deformity. Plast Reconstr Surg 1993;91(5):930–5.
24. Jacono AA, Quatela VC. Quantitative analysis of lip appearance after V-Y lip augmentation. Arch Facial Plast Surg 2004;6(3):172–7.
25. Cosman B, Gong K, Crikelair GF. Horizontal cross-lip flap with pedicle at commissure: case report. Plast Reconstr Surg 1968;41(3):273–5.
26. Rahpeyma A, Khajehahmadi S. Use of lower vermilion cross-lip flap for correction of whistle deformity in clinical practice and anatomic study for the secondary cleft lip repair. J Craniofac Surg 2013;24(4):1179–83.

27. Manafi A, Ahmadi Moghadam M, Mansouri M, et al. Repair of large lip vermilion defects with mutual cross lip musculomucosal flaps. World J Plast Surg 2012;1(1):3–10.

28. Pribaz JJ, Meara JG, Wright S, et al. Lip and vermilion reconstruction with the facial artery musculomucosal flap. Plast Reconstr Surg 2000;105(3):864–72.

29. Zarem HA, Greer DM Jr. Tongue flap for reconstruction of the lips after electrical burns. Plast Reconstr Surg 1974;53(3):310–2.

30. al-Qattan MM, Gillett D, Thomson HG. Electrical burns to the oral commissure: does splinting obviate the need for commissuroplasty? Burns 1996;22(7):555–6.

31. Garritano FG, Carr MM. Oral commissure burns in children. Oper Tech Otolaryngol Head Neck Surg 2015;26(3):136–42.

32. Su CT, Manson PN, Hoopes JE. Electrical burns of the oral commissure: treatment results and principles of reconstruction. Ann Plast Surg 1980;5(4):251–9.

33. Canady JW, Thompson SA, Bardach J. Oral commissure burns in children. Plast Reconstr Surg 1996;97(4):738–44 [discussion: 745–55].

34. Donelan MB. Reconstruction of electrical burns of the oral commissure with a ventral tongue flap. Plast Reconstr Surg 1995;95(7):1155–64.

35. Shockley WW. Scar revision techniques: z-plasty, w-plasty, and geometric broken line closure. Facial Plast Surg Clin North Am 2011;19(3):455–63.

36. Surowitz JB, Shockley WW. Enhancement of facial scars with dermabrasion. Facial Plast Surg Clin North Am 2011;19(3):517–25.

37. Sobanko JF, Alster TS. Laser treatment for improvement and minimization of facial scars. Facial Plast Surg Clin North Am 2011;19(3):527–42.

38. Castor SA, To WC, Papay FA. Lip augmentation with alloderm acellular allogenic dermal graft and fat autograft: a comparison with autologous fat injection alone. Aesthetic Plast Surg 1999;23(3):218–23.

39. Balkin DM, Samra S, Steinbacher DM. Immediate fat grafting in primary cleft lip repair. J Plast Reconstr Aesthet Surg 2014;67(12):1644–50.

40. Recupero WD, McCollough EG. Comparison of lip enhancement using autologous superficial musculoaponeurotic system tissue and postauricular fascia in conjunction with lip advancement. Arch Facial Plast Surg 2010;12(5):342–8.

41. Lassus C. Surgical vermillion augmentation: different possibilities. Aesthetic Plast Surg 1992;16(2):123–7.

42. Vecchione TR. Split vermilion grafts in reconstructive lip surgery. Br J Plast Surg 1982;35(1):67–71.

43. Ahuja RB. Vermilion reconstruction with labia minora graft. Plast Reconstr Surg 1993;92(7):1418–9.

44. Agarwal A, Gracely E, Maloney RW. Lip augmentation using sternocleidomastoid muscle and fascia grafts. Arch Facial Plast Surg 2010;12(2):97–102.

45. de Benito J, Fernandez-Sanza I. Galea and subgalea graft for lip augmentation revision. Aesthetic Plast Surg 1996;20(3):243–8.

46. Cohen SR, Kawamoto HK Jr. The free tongue graft for correction of secondary deformities of the vermilion in patients with cleft lip. Plast Reconstr Surg 1991;88(4):613–9.

47. Rohrich RJ, Reagan BJ, Adams WP Jr, et al. Early results of vermilion lip augmentation using acellular allogeneic dermis: an adjunct in facial rejuvenation. Plast Reconstr Surg 2000;105(1):409–16 [discussion: 417–8].

48. Wang J, Fan J, Nordstrom RE. Evaluation of lip augmentation with Gore-Tex facial implant. Aesthetic Plast Surg 1997;21(6):433–6.

49. San Miguel Moragas J, Reddy RR, Hernandez Alfaro F, et al. Systematic review of "filling" procedures for lip augmentation regarding types of material, outcomes and complications. J Craniomaxillofac Surg 2015;43(6):883–906.

50. Chang CS, Wallace CG, Hsiao YC, et al. Botulinum toxin to improve results in cleft lip repair: a double-blinded, randomized, vehicle-controlled clinical trial. PLoS One 2014;9(12):e115690.

51. Gassner HG, Brissett AE, Otley CC, et al. Botulinum toxin to improve facial wound healing: a prospective, blinded, placebo-controlled study. Mayo Clin Proc 2006;81(8):1023–8.

52. Wilson AM. Use of botulinum toxin type A to prevent widening of facial scars. Plast Reconstr Surg 2006;117(6):1758–66 [discussion: 1767–8].

53. Zhang DZ, Liu XY, Xiao WL, et al. Botulinum toxin type A and the prevention of hypertrophic scars on the maxillofacial area and neck: a meta-analysis of randomized controlled trials. PLoS One 2016;11(3):e0151627.

54. Gassner HG, Sherris DA, Otley CC. Treatment of facial wounds with botulinum toxin A improves cosmetic outcome in primates. Plast Reconstr Surg 2000;105(6):1948–53 [discussion: 1954–5].

55. Jablonka EM, Sherris DA, Gassner HG. Botulinum toxin to minimize facial scarring. Facial Plast Surg 2012;28(5):525–35.

56. Foo CW, Tristani-Firouzi P. Topical modalities for treatment and prevention of postsurgical hypertrophic scars. Facial Plast Surg Clin North Am 2011;19(3):551–7.

57. Mustoe TA, Cooter RD, Gold MH, et al. International clinical recommendations on scar management. Plast Reconstr Surg 2002;110(2):560–71.

58. O'Brien L, Jones DJ. Silicone gel sheeting for preventing and treating hypertrophic and keloid scars. Cochrane Database Syst Rev 2013;(9):CD003826.

59. Barr L, Barrera A. Use of hair grafting in scar camouflage. Facial Plast Surg Clin North Am 2011;19(3): 559–68.

60. Miyamoto S, Takushima A, Momosawa A, et al. Camouflaging a cleft lip scar with single-hair transplantation using a choi hair transplanter. Plast Reconstr Surg 2007;120(2):517–20.

61. Garg G, Thami GP. Micropigmentation: tattooing for medical purposes. Dermatol Surg 2005;31(8 Pt 1): 928–31 [discussion: 931].

Treating Scars in the Auricle Region

Deborah Watson, MD*, Bharat Panuganti, MD

KEYWORDS

- Auricular scar • Scar hypertrophy • Keloids • Cauliflower ear • Ear deformity

KEY POINTS

- Auricular skin does not have much laxity. Providing tensionless closure during scar repair helps minimize further scarring and ensures a favorable aesthetic result.
- Small keloids may be amenable to simple excision but larger and recurrent keloids are best managed with surgery and an adjuvant therapy.
- The cauliflower ear is often managed surgically. The most effective preventative measure is complete evacuation of the preceding auricular hematoma.

INTRODUCTION

Scarring represents an inextricable component of the healing process. From healing minor abrasions to restoring some measure of structural integrity, scarring is an inevitable outcome. Certain aesthetic and functional sequelae of scarring in the auricular region are important to understand. The external ear has inherent aesthetic value that warrants appropriate restoration during any form of reconstruction, and this has been recognized for centuries. The *Sushruta Samhita*, an ancient subcontinental Indian text, provides a description of a crude ear lobe reconstruction using a pedicled cheek flap dating back to 600 BCE.[1] Since then, enough medical and surgical experimentation has been completed to formulate treatment options for scarring in the auricular region.

RELEVANT ANATOMY AND EMBRYOLOGY

The auricle, or pinna, is the visible external component of the ear. At approximately the sixth week of gestation, the external ear develops from the proliferation of the first and second branchial arch mesenchymal cells. The tragus, helical crus, and helix are derived from the first branchial arch (Meckel cartilage). The antihelical crus, antihelix, lobule, and antitragus are derived from the second branchial arch (Reichert cartilage). The auricle reaches full adult size in many cases by 5 years of development. The external ear is formed by a framework of elastic cartilage and perichondrium with tightly adherent overlying skin, particularly over the anterior surface. The lobule is the singular noncartilaginous component, formed by a wedge of adipose tissue. The presence of only scant subcutaneous tissue necessitates careful surgical planning to preserve cosmetic auricular structure. The anterior surface of the average auricle consists of a skin envelope only 0.8 mm to 1.2 mm in thickness, firmly attached to the underlying perichondrium. In comparison, the posterior surface of the auricle bears an additional layer of fat that affords greater skin mobility and a total cumulative thickness of 1.2 mm to 3.0 mm.

BASICS OF CUTANEOUS WOUND HEALING

Scarring is an irreplaceable component of wound healing, which tends to follow a predictable

Disclosure Statement: The authors have nothing to disclose.
Division of Otolaryngology-Head and Neck Surgery, University of California, San Diego, 3350 La Jolla Village Drive, 112-C, San Diego, CA 92161, USA
* Corresponding author.
E-mail address: debwatson@ucsd.edu

Facial Plast Surg Clin N Am 25 (2017) 73–81
http://dx.doi.org/10.1016/j.fsc.2016.08.006
1064-7406/17/Published by Elsevier Inc.

pattern. Although an exhaustive explanation of the process is beyond the scope of this article, a fundamental understanding of cutaneous wound healing can shed insight on how to anticipate scarring from a therapeutic perspective.

The 3 steps of wound healing include inflammation, proliferation, and remodeling, which collectively involve a web of interactions among cytokines, vascular elements, parenchymal cells, and extracellular matrix. After tissue injury causes the disruption of blood vessels, degranulating platelets work to form a hemostatic plug and secrete wound-healing mediators, including platelet-derived growth factor (PDGF) and transforming growth factor-β (TGF-β). These growth factors are released by multiple cell types in an inactive form. Re-epithelialization of cutaneous wounds begins within hours of the initial insult, facilitated by epidermal cells migrating from skin appendages (eg, hair follicles). Wound healing continues with the formation of granulation tissue and neovascularization until fibroblasts undergo a phenotypic change to become myofibroblasts that participate in wound contraction and extracellular matrix reorganization. The transformation from granulation to scar tissue is contingent on the catabolism of collagen, which is achieved via matrix metalloproteinases. Although scarring allows the reclamation of some measure of integrity, wounds only have the opportunity to gain 20% of their final total strength within the first several weeks after the insult. Scar tissue, at maximal strength, is 70% as strong as native skin tissue.[2]

KELOIDS

Although benign in nature, keloids and hypertrophic scarring represent clinical challenges. Keloids were already recognized in ancient times as unusual tissue growth. They were referenced in the Smith papyrus from approximately 1700 BCE. The term *keloid* is derived etymologically from the Greek word, *chele*, which translates roughly to "claw of [the] crustacean," an apt reference to the tenacious grasp with which keloids resist definitive treatment.[3]

The auricular region is a well-recognized site for keloid formation after iatrogenic, incidental, or planned traumatic insult, including burns, ear piercings, and otoplasty. Keloid scarring, by definition, extends beyond the borders of the original trauma and tends to have limited prospect of natural regression (a characteristic that distinguishes it from hypertrophic scarring). It occurs with a frequency in the nonwhite population 15 times that in the white demographic.[4]

Although they remain prevalent, keloids have eluded a definitive pathophysiologic explanation. In normal skin, collagen bundles run parallel to the epithelial surface; however, types I and III collagen exist in random orientation within keloid scars. Not only is the collagen production disorganized in keloids but also it is amplified—20 times as prevalent than in normal skin.[5] Keloid formation is known to occur only in humans.[6]

Multiple theories have been postulated regarding the etiology of keloids. Several novel studies have focused on the aberrant production of various growth factors, including TGF-β and PDGF, which are involved in the chemotaxis and proliferation of keloid fibroblasts.[7] Chen and Davidson[8] report that there are low concentrations of TGB-β in the fetal wound environment, which is significantly less prone to scarring. Aberrant scar formation is also compounded by diminished synthesis of matrix metalloproteinases and higher relative apoptotic rate of normal fibroblasts compared with keloid fibroblasts.[9,10] In any case, keloid formation is likely the culmination of multiple derangements in the wound healing process.

HYPERTROPHIC SCARRING

The important clinical distinction between hypertrophic scarring and keloid is the theoretic potential for regression and the tendency to remain within the confines of the original wound. From a histologic standpoint, hypertrophic scarring consists of type III collagen bundles (apparently absent in keloids), which are oriented relatively parallel to the epithelial surface. Both types of aberrant scarring, however, are characterized by overexpression of both TGF-β and PDGF, suggesting similar pathologic derangement in the wound healing signaling process. Unlike the tendency of keloids, hypertrophic scarring has not been found more prevalent in the nonwhite population.[7]

AURICULAR HEMATOMA AND CAULIFLOWER EAR

Much like keloid scarring, auricular hematomas and their associated chondropathology are a well-recognized entity. Visual representations of the cauliflower ear, as it is known colloquially, are recorded in the annals of ancient Greek and Roman accounts as a stigmata of boxing, wrestling, and the ancient sport of pankration. The first published description of auricular hematomas as a precursor to the auricular chondropathology, was written by Bird in 1833. He described 6 cases of "inflammation of the auricle," and reported the following: "the auricle…getting hot…getting more red and even bluish" before "it will feel very hard rather soon."[11]

A more contemporary explanation for the development of the cauliflower ear is based on the result of blood collecting between the auricular perichondrium and the auricular cartilage. The blood clot essentially separates the underlying cartilage from its oxygen and nutrient source—the perichondrium. This was first recognized by Ohlsén and colleagues,[12] in which rabbit ears were injected with blood in multiple locations. Park and colleagues[13] describe their own experience with recalcitrant auricular hematomas, observing that unsuccessful management with aspiration and bolster dressings was a result of hematomas that were intracartilaginous instead. In most cases, undisturbed or residual hematomas recruit fibroblasts to create fibrosis. There also may be areas of potential neocartilage formation within the fibrotic tissue.[14] Eventually, the resultant appearance within the auricular soft tissue is one that resembles that of a cauliflower (**Fig. 1**).

In addition to being an aesthetic deformity, cauliflower ear that involves the concha can create external canal stenosis. Noormohammadpour and colleagues[15] comment on the higher incidence of audiometry-confirmed hearing loss in wrestlers affected by cauliflower ear, which is attributed to

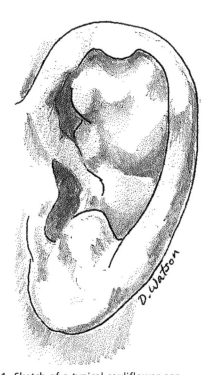

Fig. 1. Sketch of a typical cauliflower ear.

obstruction of the external auditory canal and disruption of the inherent cerumen expelling process.

SCARS FROM RHYTIDECTOMIES

Preauricular and postauricular incisions are standard for most rhyditectomy procedures. Poor wound closure technique and excess tension at the incision contribute to unsightly scars and scar widening. Scarring that results from postauricular flap necrosis after a rhytidectomy is 12.6 times likely in smokers, due to the toxic effects of nicotine on vascular supply in random-pattern flaps.[16]

To address closing tension issues across rhytidectomy incisions, Knize[17] described his experience using a force measurement instrument to quantify the force required to advance facialplasty flaps to the periauricular position, realizing that the force applied to the superficial muscular aponeurotic system flap approximates 1 kg. Similar force vector measurements were made on the same cohort of 20 ears for postauricular skin closure (approximately 0.5 kg). From his results, Knize recommended the internal splinting technique, which uses auricular cartilage as a functional anchor in 4 positions (anterior, inferior to the antitragus, superior auricular sulcus, and posterior auricular sulcus) for the facelift soft tissue advancement planes using 3-0 polyglactin sutures.[17] He suggests that the auricular cartilage can sustain up to 5 kg of force before manifesting signs of aesthetic deformity. In addition to relieving tension, the superior auricular sulcus anchor suture offers the benefit of preventing superior advancement of the temporal hairline.

MANAGEMENT AND TREATMENT
General Principles of Scar Revision

Surgical scar management, particularly in the auricular region, requires careful planning. Certain immutable guidelines govern scar creation and revision in most areas. The ideal placement of a scar, revised or not, would follow a natural skin crease or relaxed skin tension line (RSTL) to maximize imperceptibility and to minimize the tension across the wound.[18] RSTLs may not be readily apparent in youthful skin. In this situation, it may be beneficial for the clinician to ask the patient preoperatively to exaggerate facial expressions to reveal their RSTLs. In addition, proper suture technique (eg, adequate wound eversion) is an important component that helps optimize scar cosmesis. A final consideration prior to planning scar revision is timing. It is prudent to allow the normal scar an adequate amount of time to achieve its mature appearance prior to opting for surgical intervention. Hypertrophic and keloid scars, on the other hand, are candidates for earlier treatment.

Surgical Repair Options

Fusiform elliptical excision

The fusiform elliptical excision represents a simple method of scar excision, with the angles of the elliptical apices measuring 30° or less to prevent the formation of the dog-ear deformity.[19] After undermining the surrounding skin to relieve tension, multiple layers of closure are completed to accomplish adequate wound eversion (**Fig. 2**).

W-plasty scar revision

The W-plasty and the geometric broken line closure (GBLC) are methods of scar irregularization, predicated on the principle that irregular lines are less perceptible than linear scars. Both of these methods are of particular utility in scars that are not oriented parallel to RSTLs. The W-plasty technique is performed by creating opposing zigzag lines on each side of the scar and to interdigitate them during closure. Ideally, the points of the resulting W shape run parallel to RSTLs or natural skin folds. The arms of the W should be approximately 5 mm in length and angled between 60° and 90°. The surrounding tissue is undermined, and the zigzagged edges of the excised scar are reapproximated with multiple layers of closure.

Geometric line scar revision

The GBLC technique is the more exaggerated scar irregularization method preferred in longer scars typically on the face. The GBLC method entails incising a series of random geometric shapes (eg, semicircles, squares, and triangles) from one side of the scar and corresponding-shaped excisions on the contralateral edge of the scar. The excised scar is then reapproximated with a multi-layer closure.

Z-plasty scar revision

The Z-plasty technique is used to lengthen irregularly contracted scars and alter the direction of a scar that is opposed to an RSTL or natural skin crease. Although the scar acts as the common limb of the Z, 2 triangular flaps are incised and switched with each other. Geometric configurations are critical to the Z-plasty method, because the angles of the designed triangles determine the linear gains after transposition. The technique also carries the advantage of being able to realign landmark facial structures distorted by scarring (**Fig. 3**).

Wide scar excision

Wilson reports on the phenomenon of scar widening, a troubling aesthetic complication in facial scars, particularly in the periauricular region where the skin has limited laxity.[20] Scar widening occurs when distracting forces act on a suture line prior to full scar maturity, precluding the cosmetic success of even the most careful surgical

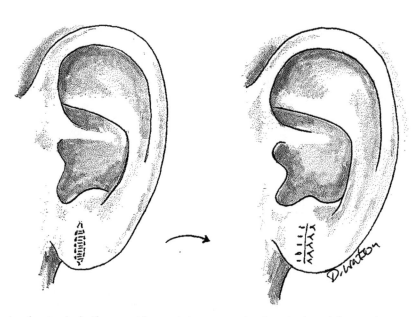

Fig. 2. Example of a simple fusiform excision and closure as a treatment of ear lobe scarring.

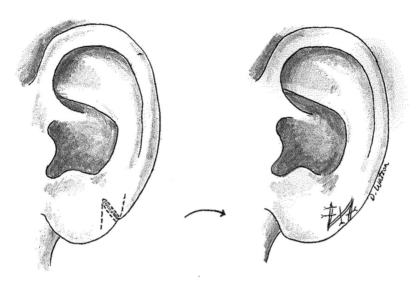

Fig. 3. Example of a Z-plasty repair for scarring and contracture of the helical rim.

wound approximation. The Millard technique, originally described in 1970, involves a split-thickness excision of scar tissue, leaving a base of scar to reduce the tension over skin. Wilson's variation on the Millard technique involves de-epithelializing the area over scar, incising the subcutaneous tissue on one side of the wound, undermining away from the incision to at least double the width of the scar, and carefully suturing the tongue of healthy native tissue over and including the extent of the tougher, underlying scar tissue.

Management for Keloids

Surgical excision

There is a plethora of literature and ongoing research describing surgical treatment protocols for keloids with varying purported efficacies. Although benign, keloid scarring resembles malignancy in its tendency toward recidivism. Froelich and colleagues[21] report that recurrence rates of keloids (the studies were not specific to auricular keloids) range between 45% and 100% when treated with surgical excision without adjuvant measures.

Kim and colleagues[22] adequately summarize a roadmap for effective surgical technique in auricular keloid resection and closure with the mnemonic, 5 As and 1 B: asepsis, atraumatic technique, absence of raw surface, avoidance of tension, accurate approximation of wound margin, and bleeding control.

Simple total (extramarginal) excision of keloid scar tends to be associated with reproliferation of keloid tissue at an incisional line closed under

tension. Therefore, Walliczek and colleagues[23] suggest using the intramarginal surgical fillet technique for auricular keloids, in which the keloid scar is sharply dissected and resected from the overlying, autoexpanded physiologic skin. The remaining native skin is then amenable to a tension-free closure.

Qi and colleagues[24] describe the X-shaped incisional method for auricular keloid removal: a cross, or X, is drawn on the keloid to guide the elevation of 4 isocentric triangular flaps from the subcutaneous tissue to preserve the vitality of the subdermal plexus and reveal the underlying keloid. The scar tissue is subsequently dissected and resected from the cartilaginous framework before the flaps are transposed and approximated with 6-0 polypropylene sutures. The study protocol included the administration of radiotherapy (900 cGy) on the first and seventh postoperative days. The average follow-up period at the time the study was published was 5.7 months, but only 1 patient reported keloid recurrence in the eleventh postoperative month.[24]

Lee and colleagues[3] describe a method of keloid core extirpation performed in 21 (Korean) patients with 24 keloids recalcitrant to nonsurgical therapy; 9 of the core excisions were performed on auricular keloids with high reported levels of patient satisfaction. In this technique, an incision is made halfway around the circumference of the keloid, 1 mm within the edge. The resulting keloid rind flap, including epidermis, dermis, and the rich subcapsular vascular plexus (located just deep to the fibrous capsule of the keloid), is raised from the fibrous keloid core. The core is subsequently extirpated leaving only a thin margin of scar tissue, before the defect is resurfaced with the aforementioned flap. The investigators reported an 87.5% nonrecurrence rate overall with a mean follow-up period of 20 months and no reported complications (eg, flap loss or congestion) in any of the auricular keloids.[3]

Ziccardi and Lamphier[25] describe the primary excision of a dumbbell-shaped ear lobe keloid, creating a large posterior lobe defect that was not amenable to cosmetic primary closure. The investigators used a full-thickness skin graft derived from the resected keloid without noted recurrence after 6 months of follow-up.[25]

The modified Chang-Park classification was developed to categorize auricular keloids by morphology (types I–V), distinguishing between pedunculated, sessile, buried, and mixed-type keloids.[26] The original Chang-Park classification was created using the same fundamental clinical criteria to make surgical approach recommendations specifically for ear lobe keloids.[27] For example, for pedunculated keloids that involve the anterior and posterior aspects of the ear lobe, a penetrating technique is used to excise the intervening lobule to reduce recurrence. For sessile-type ear lobe keloids, characterized by more horizontal growth, a wedge-resection is performed. When there is a significant lobular defect, the Z-plasty technique for closure is recommended to minimize deformity. Buried (type IV) lobular keloids present with smaller size and less pronounced contours and discoloration. The treatment recommendation is for a core excision technique, with the inclusion of both ear lobe surfaces.[27]

Adjunctive and nonsurgical therapies

Although multiple nonsurgical treatments, including silicon sheeting, intralesional steroid injections, and radiation therapy, have been purported to manage smaller auricular keloids, they are often met with unsatisfactory cosmetic results in larger keloids.

Har-Shai and colleagues[28] describe in detail the intralesional cryosurgery technique using a cryoprobe. The probe has a penetrating sealed tip that allows liquid nitrogen to be forced into its proximal end. Their data were compiled from 10 recalcitrant auricular keloids. The purported benefits included durable efficacy after a single session and a coagulative-type necrosis directed toward the keloid core, sparing the overlying melanocytes to avoid hypopigmentation.[28] Fikrle and Pizinger[29] report on their use of cryotherapy (probe or spray) in 7 patients to achieve scar volume reduction in all cases. It has been suggested

that nascent keloids are more responsive to cryotherapy.[21]

Intralesional and topical administration of chemotherapeutic agents represents a common adjunct to surgery as the primary treatment modality. Stewart and Kim[30] support the application of mitomycin C (0.4 mg/5 mL)–soaked cotton pledgets for 4 minutes after core excision of auricular keloids, reporting a 90% success rate in a 10 patient cohort followed for a mean of 8 months. The inhibition of keloid fibroblasts by mitomycin C, an antineoplastic agent that acts via alkylation to cross-link DNA, has been demonstrated in vitro to delay but not entirely inhibit the progression of fibrosis. Moreover, topical application of mitomycin has been shown to be empirically safe at a maximal concentration of 0.5 mg/5 mL.

Khare and Patil[31] report on the adjuvant administration of an alternative chemotherapeutic agent, 5-fluorouracil, injected in doses between 50 mg and 150 mg in a group of 28 patients with ear lobe keloids after surgical excision. The group attests to a recurrence rate of less than 4%, with the most common complication local tissue necrosis seen in 3 patients.[31]

Imiquimod represents an additional topical therapy that is used to attenuate keloid recurrence after resection, working as an immune-response modulator to induce interferon, interleukin, and tumor necrosis factor expression and cause fibroblast apoptosis.[32] Martín-García and Busquets[33] publish a case series, including 8 ear lobe keloids that underwent blade or electrocautery excision and daily application of 5% imiquimod cream to the resection site for 8 weeks; 50% of these keloids remained recurrence-free between 32 and 96 weeks of follow-up, whereas 6 of 8 remained recurrence-free for the 16-week observation period. As with other topical agents, untoward effects included local erythema, edema, suppuration, or ulceration.[33]

Calcium antagonism is thought to play a role in the construction of extracellular matrix. As such, intralesional verapamil is regarded as an additional adjunctive measure to minimize relapse. A case series by Lawrence[34] detailed the injection of verapamil at a concentration of 2.5 mg/mL (0.5 mL to 2.0 mL during each administration based on the size of the keloid) 7 to 14 days after surgical resection of ear lobe keloids and again 1 month after resection. Patients were also asked to wear pressure earrings. The investigator reports a 45% recurrence rate, with a greater tendency in previously treated keloids.[34]

Postoperative radiation therapy is another common therapeutic option. Ogawa and colleagues[35] analyzed 174 auricular lesions which were divided into 2 groups: 1 consisting of primary keloids and the other made up of recurrent keloids despite prior attempted surgical resection. All of the auricular keloids in their study were treated with surgery (wedge excision or simple excision ± V-Y flap for reconstruction) and postoperative radiation therapy, 10 Gy delivered in 2 fractions. The overall reported recurrence rate was 4.0%. It was suggested that the benefit of the therapy was maximal when administered within the immediate postoperative period (0–48 hours).[21]

Fruth and colleagues[36] describe the use of radiofrequency tissue volume reduction, a mechanism often used for oropharyngeal tissue in cases of obstructive sleep apnea, which functions by way of directed heating to create coagulative lesions and tissue retraction; 5 of 19 auricles were found refractory to treatment, whereas good cosmetic results were reported in 13 auricular keloids.

Steroids serve a widespread role in the treatment of primary cutaneous pathologies. Generally a 10% triamcinolone acetonide (TA) in suspension with lidocaine is injected directly into the keloid. Jung and colleagues[37] describe the use of TA as a neoadjuvant therapy, administered in doses between 0.1 mL and 1.0 mL at concentrations between 20 mg/mL and 40 mg/mL with subsequent excision of the ear lobe keloids. Injections were continued postoperatively in monthly intervals for variable total periods (2–13 total administrations) based on the clinical appearance of the lesion for a recurrence rate of 16.6% in a cohort of 18 keloids. On the other hand, Shons and Press[38] report only a single recurrence in a 31-keloid cohort treated with excision and postoperative TA injections at a mean follow-up of 35 months.

Silicone gel sheeting is a treatment option that is contingent on patient compliance. The mechanism of silicone therapy, offered in both sheet and gel formulations, on scar progression has not been ascertained. It is theorized to increase hydration of the stratum corneum and associated cytokine-mediated signaling.[39] Froelich and colleagues[39] recommend that silicone sheeting be worn as an adjuvant therapy for 12 to 24 hours a day for 2 to 12 months after definitive treatment.

Pressure therapy, often taking the form of an earring for ear lobe keloids, is an additional adjuvant therapy with minimal risk. Tanaydin and colleagues[40] report on their experience with pressure-adjustable silicone ear clips that were worn for 12 hours a day for 6 to 18 months with a recurrence rate of 29.5%. Bae-Harboe and colleagues[41] administered collagenase with adjunctive compression therapy in a cohort, including 6 ear lobe keloids. They convey that all keloids demonstrated a decrease in total size by an average of 50%, although 3 of the patients opted for surgical excision during the study.

Management of the Cauliflower Ear

The cauliflower ear is an auricular disfigurement that is often rectified surgically. The most effective preventative measure is complete evacuation of the preceding auricular hematoma.

Yotsuyanagi and colleagues[42] describe their surgical strategies for the deformity that vary based on the extent of auricular involvement. For pathology restricted to the concha, the investigators recommend an incision be made at the outer conchal margin with generous resection of the deformed cartilage to prevent recurrence. For a single-stage resection and reconstruction in cases of large cauliflower ear affecting a large portion of the ear, the investigators suggest an outer conchal incision and a post-helical incision made simultaneously for thorough cartilaginous exposure.[42] Resculpting can be accomplished carefully by scissors and/or scalpel after elevating the overlying skin, while being careful to avoid excessive injury to the underlying auricular cartilage.

Simultaneous posterior and anterior skin flaps carry the risk of devitalizing the auricle. The communicating anterior and posterior vascular plexuses of the pinna are derived primarily from the superficial temporal and posterior auricular arteries, with the most robust contribution to the middle horizontal part of the ear.[43]

Fujiwara and colleagues[44] suggest the importance of maintaining the posterior lamella of the cauliflower cartilage after resecting the anterior fibrous connective tissue, because the posterior lamella of the auricle theoretically consists of original cartilage. Contralateral conchal cartilage can be used as grafts if reconstruction is necessary to recreate any portion of the auricular framework.

Aggressive débridement of the underlying cartilage may hinder the use of full-thickness skin grafts as a reconstructive option, because of injury or loss of the perichondrium. Sutured bolsters or moldable thermal splints are useful to maintain pressure to the resection site for several months.

SUMMARY

Most auricular scarring is caused by surgical incisions and trauma; however, this region has the unique tendency to form cauliflower ear deformities as well as keloids. Many treatment options tend to be surgical in nature, but recalcitrant lesions often require a multifaceted approach with adjunctive nonsurgical therapy. The modality of treatment options is best tailored according to the type of scar and its size and location; this is especially the case for keloids. Small keloids may be amenable to simple excision, but larger and recurrent keloids are best managed with surgery and an adjuvant therapy of the clinician's choice.

Surgical management of auricular pathologies is best practiced with tension-free closure techniques. Auricular skin does not have the benefit of significant laxity compared with other regions on the face. Providing a tensionless closure is an important concept that helps to minimize scar hypertrophy, scar widening, and ensure a favorable aesthetic result. In addition, the auricular cartilaginous framework may be technically difficult to preserve. This is a prominent consideration in chondropathologies, such as the cauliflower ear, which require large areas of subcutaneous scar tissue resection. In approaching any variety of auricular scarring, all patients should be appropriately counseled regarding the risk of recurrence in keloids and nascent scar tissue in cauliflower ears. Patients should be made aware of the possibility for scar hypertrophy, widening of the scar, and persisting contour deformities.

REFERENCES

1. Weerda H. History of auricular reconstruction. Adv Otorhinolaryngol 2010;68:1–24. Available at: http://www.karger.com/Article/Abstract/314560. Accessed March 1, 2016.
2. Epstein FH, Singer AJ, Clark RA. Cutaneous wound healing. N Engl J Med 1999;341(10):738–46.
3. Lee Y, Minn K-W, Baek R-M, et al. A new surgical treatment of keloid: keloid core excision. Ann Plast Surg 2001;46(2):135–40.
4. Su C, Alizadeh K, Boddie A, et al. The problem scar. Clin Plast Surg 1998;25(3):451–65.
5. Rockwell WB, Cohen I, Ehrlich H. Keloids and hypertrophic scars: a comprehensive review. Plast Reconstr Surg 1989;84(5):827–37.
6. Chike-Obi C, Cole P, Brissett A. Keloids: pathogenesis, clinical features, and management. Semin Plast Surg 2009;23(03):178–84.
7. Wolfram D, Tzankov A, Pülzl P, et al. Hypertrophic scars and keloids—a review of their pathophysiology, risk factors, and therapeutic management. Dermatol Surg 2009;35(2):171–81.
8. Chen MA, Davidson TM. Scar management: prevention and treatment strategies. Curr Opin Otolaryngol Head Neck Surg 2005;13(4):242–7.
9. Niessen F, Spauwen P, Schalkwijk J, et al. On the nature of hypertrophic scars and keloids: a review. Plast Reconstr Surg 1999;104(5):1435–58.
10. Luo S, Benatham M, Raffoul W, et al. Abnormal balance between proliferation and apoptotic cell death in fibroblasts derived from keloid lesions. Plast Reconstr Surg 2001;107(1):87–96.
11. Mudry A, Pirsig W. Auricular hematoma and cauliflower deformation of the ear: from art to medicine. Otol Neurotol 2009;30(1):116–20.
12. Ohlsén L, Skoog T, Sohn SA. The pathogenesis of cauliflower ear: an experimental study in rabbits. Scand J Plast Reconstr Surg 1975;9(1):34–9.
13. Ghanem T, Rasamny JK, Park SS. Rethinking auricular trauma. Laryngoscope 2005;115(7):1251–5.
14. Roy S, Smith LP. A novel technique for treating auricular hematomas in mixed martial artists (ultimate fighters). Am J Otolaryngol 2010;31(1): 21–4.
15. Noormohammadpour P, Rostami M, Nourian R, et al. Association between hearing loss and cauliflower ear in wrestlers, a case control study employing hearing tests. Asian J Sports Med 2015;6(2): e25786.
16. Adamson P, Moral M. Complications of cervicofacial rhytidectomy. Facial Plast Surg Clin North Am 1993; 112:257–70.
17. Knize D. Periauricular face lift incisions and auricular anchor. Plast Reconstr Surg 1999;104(5):1508–14.
18. Lee KK, Mehrany K, Swanson NA. Surgical revision. Dermatol Clin 2005;23(1):141–50.
19. Watson D, Reuther M. Scar revision techniques—pearls and pitfalls. Facial Plast Surg 2012;28(05): 487–91.
20. Wilson A. Widening of scars: foe coaxed into a friend? The Millard technique revisited. Plast Reconstr Surg 2000;106(7):1488–93.
21. Froelich K, Staudenmaier R, Kleinsasser N, et al. Therapy of auricular keloids: review of different treatment modalities and proposal for a therapeutic algorithm. Eur Arch Otorhinolaryngol 2007;264(12): 1497–508.
22. Kim DY, Kim ES, Eo SR, et al. A surgical approach for earlobe keloid: keloid fillet flap. Plast Reconstr Surg 2004;113(6):1668–74.
23. Walliczek U, Engel S, Weiss C, et al. Clinical outcome and quality of life after a multimodal therapy approach to ear keloids. JAMA Facial Plast Surg 2015;17(5):333–9.
24. Qi Z, Liang W, Wang Y, et al. "X"-shaped incision and keloid skin-flap resurfacing: a new surgical method for auricle keloid excision and reconstruction. Dermatol Surg 2012;38(8):1378–82.
25. Ziccardi VB, Lamphier J. Use of keloid skin as an autograft for earlobe reconstruction after excision. Oral Surg Oral Med Oral Pathol Oral Radiol Endod 2000;89(6):674–5.
26. Park SY, Lee G-H, Park JM, et al. Clinical characteristics of auricular keloids treated with surgical excision. Korean J Audiol 2012;16(3):134.
27. Park TH, Seo SW, Kim JK, et al. Earlobe keloids: classification according to gross morphology

Determines proper surgical approach. Dermatol Surg 2012;38(3):406–12.

28. Har-Shai Y, Ravagnani PM, Galli S, et al. Intralesional cryosurgery enhances the involution of recalcitrant auricular keloids: a new clinical approach supported by experimental studies. Wound Repair Regen 2006;14(1):18–27.

29. Fikrle T, Pizinger K. Cryosurgery in the treatment of earlobe keloids: report of seven cases. Dermatol Surg 2005;31(12):1728–31.

30. Stewart CE 4th, Kim J. Application of mitomycin-C for head and neck keloids. Otolaryngol Head Neck Surg 2006;135(6):946–50.

31. Khare N, Patil SB. A novel approach for management of ear keloids: Results of excision combined with 5-fluorouracil injection. J Plast Reconstr Aesthet Surg 2012;65(11):e315–7.

32. Jacob SE, Berman B, Nassiri M, et al. Topical application of imiquimod 5% cream to keloids alters expression genes associated with apoptosis. Br J Dermatol 2003;149(Suppl 66):62–5.

33. Martín-García RF, Busquets AC. Postsurgical use of imiquimod 5% cream in the prevention of earlobe keloid recurrences: results of an open-label, pilot study. Dermatol Surg 2005;31(11 Pt 1):1394–8.

34. Lawrence WT. Treatment of earlobe keloids with surgery plus adjuvant intralesional verapamil and pressure earrings. Ann Plast Surg 1996;37(2):167–9.

35. Ogawa R, Huang C, Akaishi S, et al. Analysis of surgical treatments for earlobe keloids: analysis of 174 lesions in 145 patients. Plast Reconstr Surg 2013; 132(5):818e–25e.

36. Fruth K, Gouveris H, Kuelkens C, et al. Radiofrequency tissue volume reduction for treatment of auricle keloids. Laryngoscope 2011;121(6):1233–6.

37. Jung JY, Roh MR, Kwon YS, et al. Surgery and perioperative intralesional corticosteroid injection for treating earlobe keloids: a Korean experience. Ann Dermatol 2009;21(3):221–5.

38. Shons A, Press B. The treatment of earlobe keloids by surgical excision and postoperative triamcinolone injection. Ann Plast Surg 1983;10(6):480–2.

39. Mustoe T. Evolution of silicone therapy and mechanism of action in scar management. Aesthetic Plast Surg 2008;32(1):82–92.

40. Tanaydin V, Beugels J, Piatkowski A, et al. Efficacy of custom-made pressure clips for ear keloid treatment after surgical excision. J Plast Reconstr Aesthet Surg 2016;69(1):115–21.

41. Bae-Harboe Y-SC, Harboe-Schmidt JE, Graber E, et al. Collagenase followed by compression for the treatment of earlobe keloids. Dermatol Surg 2014; 40(5):519–24.

42. Yotsuyanagi T, Yamashita K, Urushidate S, et al. Surgical correction of cauliflower ear. Br J Plast Surg 2002;55(5):380–6.

43. Atamaz Pinar Y, Asli Aktan Ikiz Z, Bilge O. Arterial anatomy of the auricle: its importance for reconstructive surgery. Surg Radiol Anat 2003;25(3–4): 175–9.

44. Fujiwara M, Suzuki A, Nagata T, et al. Cauliflower ear dissection. J Plast Reconstr Aesthet Surg 2011; 64(11):e279–82.

Treatment of Scalp Scars

John Kim[a,b,*]

KEYWORDS

• Scalp • Reconstruction • Scar • Defect • Anatomy

KEY POINTS

- The scalp has unique features that must be taken into consideration when planning reconstruction of defects or revision of scars.
- The reconstructive surgeon must be familiar with the unique anatomic features of the scalp when considering surgical problems of the scalp.
- The reconstructive surgeon should consider the reconstructive options commonly referred to as the reconstructive ladder when approaching surgical problems of the scalp.

The scalp is a visible portion of the anatomy that provides both a cosmetic and functional challenge when considering reconstruction and scar revision. The scalp provides a covering for the calvarium. It contains hair follicles that form the basis of hair and hairstyles. "Hair today, gone tomorrow," refers to the challenge of the possibility of the changing hairscape over time. This change must also be considered when considering reconstruction or scar revision of the scalp. These factors must be considered both when creating and revising a scar to the scalp. The unique nature of the scalp offers many challenges and requires the reconstructive surgeon to be versatile to achieve a successful reconstruction.

ANATOMY OF THE SCALP

In reconstructing any regional anatomic site, it is important to be well-versed in the anatomy of the region. Any discussion on the anatomy of the scalp will likely include the familiar mnemonic SCALP. This mnemonic stands for Skin, subCutaneous tissue, galea Aponeurotica, Loose areolar tissue, and Pericranium. The skin layer can be quite thick, up to 8 mm in some areas.[1,2] The follicles are also contained in the skin layer and in the subcutaneous layer and provide a unique challenge to scar revision. The vascular supply of the scalp, lymphatics, and nerves are largely contained within the subcutaneous tissue. The galea aponeurotica provides a tough layer of connective tissue that can be used as an anchor layer to hold tension with reconstruction. The galea aponeurotica is contiguous with the fascia of the frontalis muscle anteriorly and the occipitalis muscle posteriorly. Laterally, the galea aponeurotica is contiguous with the temporoparietal fascia. One important consideration is the fusion of the galea aponeurotica with the pericranium at the linea temporalis especially at the frontal lateral region.[3] The loose connective tissue under the galea aponeurotica provides the scalp with a significant amount of mobility. The pericranium or the periosteum of the calvarium is tightly adherent to the underlying bone. This final layer of scalp is important for reconstruction if a vascularized layer is required for receipt of a skin graft or healing by secondary intention.

The temporal aspect of the scalp presents a few important points worth reviewing. The skin and subcutaneous tissue is similar to the scheme as described. The galea aponeurotic, however, fuses with the temporoparietal fascia in this region. As mentioned, the galea aponeurotica is contiguous with the fascia of the frontalis muscle anteriorly and the occipitalis muscle posteriorly. Also of interest, the temporoparietal fascia is contiguous with the superficial musculoaponeurotic system inferiorly. The frontal branch of the facial nerve

a Kaiser Permanente, SC, USA; b 10800 Magnolia Avenue, Riverside, CA 92505, USA
* 10800 Magnolia Avenue, Riverside, CA 92505.
E-mail address: joki777@hotmail.com

Facial Plast Surg Clin N Am 25 (2017) 83–88
http://dx.doi.org/10.1016/j.fsc.2016.08.013

and the superficial temporal artery are found within the temporoparietal fascia.[4] Underneath the temporoparietal fascia can be found the familiar loose areolar connective tissue similar to the corresponding layer found under the galea aponeurotica. There may be some confusion as to the name of the temporoparietal fascia, because it is sometimes referred to as the superficial temporal fascia. The temporalis fascia, also referred to as the deep temporal fascia, can be found deep to the loose areolar tissue. The temporalis fascia (or deep temporal fascia) is noted to form a superficial and deep layer as it surrounds the superficial temporal fat pad approximately 2 to 3 cm superior to the zygomatic arch. The temporoparietal fascia and the superficial layer of the temporalis fascia (or deep temporal fascia) and periosteum of the zygomatic arch become a quasi fusion of dense connective tissue at the level of the zygomatic arch. The frontal branch of the facial nerve is generally found to cross the zygomatic arch at the middle third of the zygomatic arch and it is at the level of the arch that the nerve is at particular risk for injury given this condensation of layers.

The vascular supply to the scalp is a rich network of vessels supplied by the internal and external carotid arteries as well as the terminal branches originating from the subclavian artery and, in small part, the dorsal branches of the posterior intercostal arteries. This network of vessels has broad anastomosis that allow for vascularization of the entire network with 1 or more branches.[5–7] The anterior scalp vascular supply is through the supraorbital and supratrochlear arteries that arise from the ophthalmic artery originating from the internal carotid artery. The posterior supply is from separate sources depending on whether the region in question is above or below the nuchal line. In general, the arterial supply above the nuchal line is from the occipital artery, which is a terminal branch of the external carotid artery. Below the nuchal line, the scalp receives arterial supply from the musculocutaneous perforators of the splenius capitus and trapezius muscles. These originate from the dorsal branches of the posterior intercostal arteries and a branch of the transverse cervical artery respectively. There is a relatively small contribution to the postauricular area of the scalp by the postauricular artery, another terminal branch of the external carotid artery.

Lymphatic drainage of the scalp is found in the subcutaneous layer and in large part follows the venous drainage. This drainage pattern is highly variable and can be seen to drain to the parotid, postauricular, suboccipital, posterior cervical, and jugulodigastric lymph nodes.[8–10]

Anterior and lateral sensory innervation is provided through the branches of the trigeminal nerve by way of the supraorbital, supratrochlear, zygomaticotemporal, and auriculotemporal nerves. The supraorbital and supratrochlear nerves supply sensation anteriorly. The zygomaticotemporal and auriculotemproal nerves supply sensation laterally. Posterior sensory innervation is supplied by the greater and lesser occipital nerves. These nerves originate from the dorsal rami of the cervical spinal nerves and the cervical plexus.

ANATOMY OF THE FOLLICLE

A complete presentation of the anatomy of the hair follicle is complex and is beyond the scope of this paper. Important to our discussion of scar revision of the scalp, the hair follicle contains the sebaceous unit and the bulb within the dermal and subcutaneous portion of the scalp, respectively. The bulb extends down to the subcutaneous tissue. The orientation of the follicle in the dermis and subcutaneous tissue is an important consideration in the creation of the incision into the scalp skin. The preservation of the bulb and the sebaceous unit is important to maximize the chances of survival of the follicle and retain the ability of hair growth.

Scars or defects to the scalp may be a result of multiple etiologies including congenital lesions; excision of benign or malignant lesions; thermal, electrical, or chemical burns; various forms of alopecia; trauma; and radiation. Although this list is not exhaustive, it underscores the point that the causes of scalp scar are many. Clearly, the size and location of the scar will influence the options for reconstruction. When considering reconstruction of the scalp or revision of scars to the scalp, the reconstructive surgeon must consider the reconstructive ladder.

SECONDARY INTENTION

Secondary intention is a viable option for defects of the scalp. The advantages include the elimination of surgery for the nonsurgical or poor surgical candidate. The disadvantages include loss of hair, poor texture, and color and contour match of the final result. The length of time for healing is another disadvantage. Although a vascularized layer is obviously helpful, few authors have reported excellent success with tissue coverage, even with fairly large defects involving exposed bone without pericranium. One retrospective study reported a series of 38 patients with exposed bone with a mean area of exposed bone measuring 107.4 cm^2. The mean time to epithelialization of the area of exposed bone was 13 weeks. The authors concluded that healing by secondary intention was a viable and safe option for treatment of scalp defects with bone exposure on selected patients.[11] The postradiation patient is not a good candidate for healing by secondary intention if bone exposure is encountered.

PRIMARY CLOSURE

Primary closure is considered the preferred method of closure if primary closure can be achieved given the size of the defect. In general, defects that have dimensions of 3 cm or less seem to be most amenable to primary closure. Certainly, closure of defects with greater dimensions have been reported, but these generally involve the loose areas of the scalp that overlie muscle. Care must be taken to place the tension on the galeal layer. Relaxing incisions to the galea aponeurotica may be made perpendicular to the direction of closure. These relaxing incision may be made approximately 2 cm apart, keeping in mind that the vascular supply of the scalp lies in the plane above the galea. Even with the relaxing incisions, the amount of tissue mobility may be limited. Advantages to primary closure include relatively fast recovery time, maintaining hair-bearing skin, good contour, and color and texture match. The disadvantages include the limited size of defects that can be closed and alopecia owing to increased skin tension with tight closures.

SKIN GRAFT

For defects too large for primary closure, skin grafts offer an advantage of allowing for coverage of larger surface areas. Disadvantages include relatively poor color, contour, and texture match, as well as loss of hair-bearing tissue. Healing time is relatively longer when taking into account the length of time to achieve stabilized results. Full-thickness skin grafts have the advantage of less donor site morbidity and improved cosmetic outcome as compared with split thickness skin grafts. Split thickness skin grafts give the advantage of availability of greater surface areas. Popular donor sites for full-thickness skin grafts to the scalp include the neck, abdomen, groin, upper arm, inner thigh, and buttocks. As opposed to healing by secondary intention, having vascularized tissue is essential for placement of skin grafts. If bone exposure is present, an option may to delay the skin graft and drill holes into the outer cortex to allow for granulation. This technique can be fraught with complications, including delay of granulation, poor contour match, and ultimate loss of epithelial coverage.

LOCAL FLAPS

Local flaps are available for closure of defects and can be useful for closure of some defects that are not amenable to primary closure. These local flaps are limited in that closure of defects with diameters of greater than 6 cm become exceedingly difficult to close. Consideration must be given to the placement of incisions, so as, as much as possible, not to expose incisions beyond hair-bearing skin. Rotational flaps are generally of more use than advancement flaps given the lack of elasticity of the scalp. In general, it is recommended that incisions for rotational flaps be 4 to 6 times the length of the defect to maximize the extension of the flap. Among various described local flaps, the multirotational flap is a classically described flap for the closure of medium sized defects to the scalp.[12–14]

One option that can be useful is to use a combination of both local flaps and skin grafts. This approach may be useful for medium to large defects involving exposed bone. Although the exposed bone may be covered with a pericranial flap for the purpose of accepting a skin graft,[15] this method may not be successful in that the recipient site of the skin graft may be tenuous. Instead, a local flap consisting of the layers including the skin down to and including the galea may be used to close the defect involving the exposed bone. The donor site, with the periosteum left undisturbed, can be reconstructed with a skin graft.

REGIONAL FLAPS

Regional flaps have been described for the use of closure of large defects to the scalp. Generally, these flaps are used for the patient who may not tolerate free tissue transfer with vascular anastomosis. The classically described flaps include the lower island trapezius flap and the latissimus dorsi musculocutaneous flap.[16–19] These flaps have the disadvantage of poor cosmetic results secondary to the bulky nature of the flaps and the tension along the pedicle of the flaps. They do have the advantage of providing large amounts of vascularized tissue for coverage of large scalp defects.

TISSUE EXPANSION

When more donor tissue is required, tissue expansion can be accomplished to a limited degree during intraoperative reconstruction. This technique involves placing the tissue on stretch intraoperatively to achieve mechanical expansion, which depends on stretching existing tissue and realignment of collagen bundles by acute stress.[20]

Controlled tissue expansion can also be achieved with the use of internal tissue expanders that are placed either before the excision of a lesion or after the excision once the wound has stabilized. Tissue expansion results in biological creep, which produces cellular proliferation secondary to slow sustained stress. Microscopically, this results in increased epidermal thickness and transient dermal thinning.[20] When placing the tissue expanders, the base of the tissue expander is recommended to be 2.5 times the area of the defect.[21] It is not recommended to place tissue expanders in previously irradiated skin.[22] Advantages to the use of tissue expanders in reconstruction of scalp defects include good color, texture, and contour match and ability to bring in hair bearing tissue. The density of hair is decreased in comparison with nonexpanded skin; however, the difference may not be noticeable to the observer unless the expansion is carried out to the extreme. Timing and time is also a factor in the decision to proceed with tissue expansion. The tissue expansion may well take weeks to complete. The expansion can also result in erosion or infection of the donor skin, which may make the situation worse.

FREE TISSUE TRANSFER

For the patient who is able to tolerate a larger reconstruction, the free tissue transfer with vascular anastomosis offers the advantage of providing large amounts of vascularized tissue with the advantage of being able to achieve superior cosmetic results when compared with regional flaps. These flaps are useful for instances of large scalp defects, in previously irradiated tissue, or to cover large areas of alloplastic material. The disadvantages include the increased operative time and complexity of the procedure, which some patients may not be able to tolerate medically. Obviously, the color and texture match is poor, but the contour can be refined and has the potential to be adequate. Of course, the flap will not bring hair bearing skin that can pass for scalp hair. Multiple flaps have been described for reconstruction of the scalp including the latissimus dorsi flap, radial forearm, anterolateral thigh, gracillis, lateral arm, parascapular, rectus abdominis, scarp adipofascial, and omental flaps.[22–32]

FOLLICULAR UNIT TRANSPLANTS

Historically, hair transplantation has been used with some success for treatment of scalp scars.[4,33–35] Current techniques with follicular unit transplants may be useful to camouflage scars.[36,37] They are not considered useful for areas of hair loss previously reconstructed with skin graft or where there is loss of subcutaneous tissue.

GENERAL CONSIDERATIONS FOR SCALP SCAR REVISION

Although many options may be used for any given defect, there are some general considerations for scalp scar revision.

Location

Does the defect involve non–hair-bearing or hair-bearing scalp or both? Will the placement of incisions be a factor because of the location of the defect? Will the reconstruction ideally involve replacing tissue with hair bearing skin?

Size

How large is the defect and can it be closed with primary closure or a local flap? Larger defects may require a skin graft, tissue expansion, or a local regional flap or free tissue transfer.

Hair or No Hair

Scars to the non–hair-bearing scalp can be a challenge owing to the exposed nature of the scar; however, scar revisions to the hair-bearing region of the scalp can present another challenge in that reconstruction ideally would include replacing the scar with hair-bearing tissue. This may not always be possible given the size and location of the defect. Future hair loss should also be considered when planning reconstruction of the scalp. This is important in terms of planning incisions that may become more visible with hair loss or reconstructive options that may be more attractive when taking into consideration future hair loss.

Exposed Bone

As mentioned, bone exposure can limit the options on the reconstructive ladder. As stated, a useful option may be to use a combination of the local flap and skin graft.

Prior or Planned Future Radiation

Radiation can greatly increase the complication rates and will limit the usefulness of many of the options in the reconstructive ladder.

Direction of Incision Through Hair-bearing Skin

When making incisions through hair-bearing skin, the incision should be beveled to parallel the direction of the follicles in the region so as to minimize trauma to the follicles. Great care should be taken to minimize transection of the follicle with the goal to preserve both the bulb and sebaceous unit of the follicle. Minimizing cautery to the skin and subcutaneous layer is also key to minimizing damage to the follicles.

Medical Comorbidities

Can the patient tolerate the proposed reconstruction? Certainly, the greater the comorbidity, the more limited the options may be on the reconstructive ladder.

SUMMARY

The scalp presents many challenges to the reconstructive surgeon given its visible nature and the various considerations that must be given for optimal reconstruction. In this article, we have reviewed the anatomy of the scalp, the various options for reconstruction and important considerations for improving the chances of optimal reconstruction of scalp defects.

REFERENCES

1. Reund RM. Scalp, calvarium and forehead reconstruction. In: Aston SJ, Beasley RW, Thorne CHM, editors. Grabb and Smith's plastic surgery. Philadelphia: Lippincott-Raven; 1997. p. 473.
2. Shestak KC, Ramasastry SS. Reconstruction of defects of the scalp and skull. In: Cohen M, editor. Mastery of plastic and reconstructive surgery. Boston: Little, Brown; 1994. p. 830–41.
3. Moss CJ, Menelson BC, Taylor GI. Surgical anatomy of the ligamentous attachments in the temple and periorbital regions. Plast Reconstr Surg 2000; 105(4):1475–90.
4. Hoffmann JF. Reconstruction of the scalp. In: Baker SR, editor. Local flaps in facial reconstruction. St Louis (MO): Mosby; 2007. p. 638.
5. Nasir S, Karaaltin M, Erdem A. Total scalp replantation: surgical tricks and pitfalls. J Craniofac Surg 2015;26(4):1192–5.
6. Miller GD, Anstee EJ, Snell JA. Successful replantation of an avulsed scalp by microvascular anastomoses. Plast Reconstr Surg 1976;58(2):133–6.
7. Kaplan HY, Yaffe B, Borenstein A. Single artery replantation of totally avulsed scalp. Injury 1993;24(7):488–90.
8. Cappello ZJ, Augenstein AC, Potts KL, et al. Sentinel lymph node status is the most important prognostic factor in patients with melanoma of the scalp. Laryngoscope 2013;123(6):1411–5.
9. Monroe MM, Pattisapu P, Myers JN, et al. Sentinel lymph node biopsy provides prognostic value in thick head and neck melanoma. Otolaryngol Head Neck Surg 2015;153(3):372–8.
10. Close LG, Goepfert H, Ballantyne AJ, et al. Malignant melanoma of the scalp. Laryngoscope 1979; 89(8):1189–96.
11. Becker GD, Adams LA, Levin BC. Secondary intention healing of exposed scalp and forehead bone after Mohs surgery. Otolaryngol Head Neck Surg 1999;121(6):751–4.
12. Moulton-Barrett R, Vanderschelden B. Double-opposing unilobar rotation flaps in the reconstruction of moderate-to-large defects of the scalp. J Craniofac Surg 2015;26(6):e523–5.
13. Orticochea M. Four flap scalp reconstruction technique. Br J Plast Surg 1967;20(2):159–71.
14. Orticochea M. New three-flap reconstruction technique. Br J Plast Surg 1971;24(2):184–8.
15. Terranova W. The use of periosteal flaps in scalp and forehead reconstruction. Ann Plast Surg 1990;25(6): 450–6.
16. Uğurlu K, Özçelik D, Hüthüt I, et al. Extended vertical trapezius myocutaneous flap in head and neck reconstruction as a salvage procedure. Plast Reconstr Surg 2004;114(2):339–50.
17. Lynch JR, Hansen JE, Chaffoo R, et al. The lower trapezius musculocutaneous flap revisited: versatile coverage for complicated wounds to the posterior cervical and occipital regions based on the deep branch of the transverse cervical artery. Plast Reconstr Surg 2002;109(2):444–50.
18. Tanaka Y, Miki K, Tajima S, et al. Reconstruction of an extensive scalp defect using the split latissimus dorsi flap in combination with the serratus anterior musculoosseous flap. Br J Plast Surg 1998;51(3):250–4.
19. Har-El G, Bhaya M, Sundaram K. Latissimus dorsi myocutaneous flap for secondary head and neck reconstruction. Am J Otolaryngol 1999;20(5): 287–93.
20. Cox AJ III, Wang TD, Cook TA. Closure of a scalp defect. Arch Facial Plast Surg 1999;1(3):212–5.
21. Baker SR, Swanson NA. Tissue expansion of the head and neck: indications technique, and complications. Arch Otolaryngol Head Neck Surg 1990; 116(10):1147–53.
22. Hussussian CJ, Reece GP. Microsurgical scalp reconstruction in the patient with cancer. Plast Reconstr Surg 2002;109(6):1828–34.
23. Newman MI, Hanasono MM, Disa JJ, et al. Scalp reconstruction: a 15-year experience. Ann Plast Surg 2004;52(5):501–6.
24. Borah GL, Hidalgo DA, Wey PD. Reconstruction of extensive scalp defects with rectus free flaps. Ann Plast Surg 1995;34(3):281–5.

25. Lutz BS. Aesthetic and functional advantages of the anterolateral thigh flap in reconstruction of tumor-related scalp defects. Microsurgery 2002;22(6):258–64.

26. Ikuta Y. Microvascular free transfer of omentum. In: Vasconez LO, Strauch B, editors. Grabb's encyclopedia of flaps. 2nd edition. Philadelphia: Lippincott-Raven; 1998. p. 42–4.

27. Wax MK, Burkey BB, Bascom D, et al. The role of free tissue transfer in the reconstruction of massive neglected skin cancers of the head and neck. Arch Facial Plast Surg 2003;5(6):479–82.

28. Lee B, Bickel K, Levin S. Microsurgical reconstruction of extensive scalp defects. J Reconstr Microsurg 1999;15(4):255–62.

29. Lutz BS, Wei FC, Chen HC, et al. Reconstruction of scalp defects with free flaps in 30 cases. Br J Plast Surg 1998;51(3):186–90.

30. Pennington DG, Stern HS, Lee KK. Free-flap reconstruction of large defects of the scalp and calvarium. Plast Reconstr Surg 1989;83(4):655–61.

31. Chicarilli ZN, Ariyan S, Cuono CB. Single-stage repair of complex scalp and cranial defects with the free radial forearm flap. Plast Reconstr Surg 1986;77(4):577–85.

32. Koshima I, Inagawa K, Jitsuiki Y, et al. Scarpa's adipofascial flap repair of wide scalp defects. Ann Plast Surg 1996;36(1):88–92.

33. Barrera A. The use of micrografts and minigrafts for the treatment of burn alopecia. Plast Reconstr Surg 1999;103(2):581–4.

34. Nordström RE. Punch hair grafting under split-skin grafts on scalps. Plast Reconstr Surg 1979;64(1):9–12.

35. Limmer BL, Buchwach KA. Hair transplantation using follicular unit micrografting. Facial Plast Surg 1999;7(4):523–35.

36. Jung S, Oh SJ, Hoon Koh S. Hair follicle transplantation on scar tissue. J Craniofac Surg 2013;24(4):1239–41.

37. Barr L, Barrera A. Use of hair grafting in scar camouflage. Facial Plast Surg Clin North Am 2011;19(3):559–68.

Treating Scars on the Oral Mucosa

Erik William Evans, DDS, MD

KEYWORDS

• Mucosa • Scar • Skin • Fibroblast • Epithelium • TGF-β • Wound

KEY POINTS

- Oral mucosal scars are not as functionally or aesthetically significant as facial skin scars.
- Oral mucosa heals faster and with less scarring than skin mainly due to differences in fibroblast, macrophage, and neutrophil activity at various stages of wound healing.
- Surgical wounding of oral mucosa results in minimal scarring; however, the unique anatomy of the oral cavity makes planning surgical incisions and closure imperative.
- Traumatic and ablative wounds of the oral mucosa are more easily reconstructed than facial skin wounds due to the mobility of mucosa, minimal scarring, and the decreased aesthetic exposure as compared with the skin of the face.
- Mucosal tissue, specifically buccal mucosa, serves as a predictable donor tissue for reconstruction of soft tissue defects, most commonly the urethra.

INTRODUCTION

Wound healing results in a variable amount of scar formation. The resulting scar's impact on function and aesthetics is greatest on the skin. Mucosal wounds tend to heal more rapidly than skin wounds and with minimal to no scar formation and hence have minimal impact on function or aesthetics.

Most mucous membranes exist throughout the body and serve in various functions, the anatomy of which varies based on its function in that location. Mucosa serves as the epithelial barrier in the gastrointestinal, genitourinary, and respiratory systems. Due to the varied nature of the structure and function of mucosal barriers throughout the body as well as the intent of this text, the focus of this article is scars of the oral cavity mucosa. Inferences may be made to the stratified squamous mucosa of the ocular conjunctiva due to its similar histology and the common scarring diseases (ie, cicatricle pemphigoid) that may affect both oral mucosa and conjunctiva.

Mucosa differs from skin in its anatomy as well as its relatively diminished propensity to scar. Given this fact and its relative lack of aesthetic significance as compared with the facial skin, the necessity of treatment of scars to the mucosa is minimal. However, a review of the differences in the anatomy, physiology, and behavior of mucosa from skin, diseases manifested in mucosa, and the management of incisions and traumatic injuries to mucosa is presented.

ANATOMY AND FUNCTION

The oral cavity is lined with a continuous layer of mucous membrane that is contiguous with the skin at the vermillion border of the lips and the pharyngeal mucosa. It is predominantly of

Disclosures: None.
Division of Oral and Maxillofacial Surgery, University of Cincinnati Medical Center, Veterans Affairs Medical Center, Cincinnati Children's Hospital Medical Center, 200 Albert Sabin Way, ML 0461, Cincinnati, OH 45219, USA
E-mail address: Erik.evans@uc.edu

Facial Plast Surg Clin N Am 25 (2017) 89–97
http://dx.doi.org/10.1016/j.fsc.2016.08.008
1064-7406/17/© 2016 Elsevier Inc. All rights reserved.

ectodermal origin and consists of keratinized and nonkeratinized stratified squamous epithelium.

The specialized mucosa of the dorsal surface of the tongue contains a multitude of epithelial papillae. The lips, cheeks, vestibules, floor of mouth, and ventral tongue consist of lining mucosa (**Fig. 1**). It has minimal function in mastication and is soft, pliable, and its surface is nonkeratinized epithelium (**Fig. 2**). The hard palate and gingiva consist of masticatory, or attached, mucosa of keratinized epithelium and have a greater function in mastication.

Like skin, the functions of mucosa are to serve as a protective barrier to mechanical and microbiologic insults; sensation to temperature, touch, and pain; and secretion. The thinness of the floor of mouth mucosa also allows for rapid absorption of medications.

The anatomy of both skin and mucosa are similar. They both contain structurally similar layers. Some nomenclature differs between skin and mucosal histology, such as the dermis of skin is equivalent to the lamina propria of mucosa. The histologic differences between keratinized mucosa, nonkeratinized mucosa, and skin may be seen in **Fig. 3**.

Skin Versus Mucosa

Epithelial wounds invariably end in scar formation. Cutaneous scars range from having little or no impact on function and aesthetics to hypertrophic scars or contractures that may interfere with function and aesthetics. The steps of the healing process are similar in both skin and mucosal wounds. However, it has been said that healing of mucosal wounds is akin to that of fetal tissues, with rapid remodeling and minimal scar formation in comparison with wounds of the skin[1] (**Fig. 4**). In

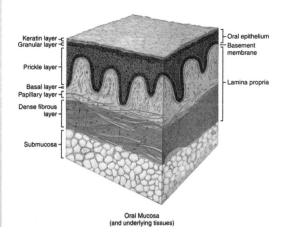

Keratin layer
Granular layer
Oral epithelium
Basement membrane
Prickle layer
Basal layer
Papillary layer
Lamina propria
Dense fibrous layer
Submucosa

Oral Mucosa
(and underlying tissues)

Fig. 1. Schematic of layers of oral mucosa.

comparison with skin wounds, mucosal wounds exhibit a lower inflammatory response with lower neutrophil, macrophage, and T-cell infiltration, as well as decreased expression of proinflammatory TGF-β_1.[2,3]

Environmental differences also exist between skin and mucosa, such as moisture, as a result of salivary flow and microflora. However, histologic studies of skin transposed into the oral cavity show that skin maintains its morphologic characteristics after transplantation.[4] This is clearly seen after the inset of regional or distant cutaneous flaps into the oral cavity with the continuation of hair growth and, in one reported case, the formation of a keloid. These findings imply that the repair in oral mucosa is likely to involve intrinsic characteristics of mucosal tissue and is not only due to environmental factors.

Transforming growth factor-β (TGF-β), and more specifically, the TGF-β_1 isoform, is activated in the wound-repair process and promotes inflammatory cell recruitment. Platelets release TGF-β_1 immediately after injury, which recruit collagen-producing fibroblasts. Inflammatory cells continue to produce TGF-β_1 throughout all stages of wound healing. Due to its proinflammatory properties, TGF-β_1 has been implicated as an important factor in scar formation as well as hypertrophic scars and keloids. Studies have shown decreased TGF-β_1 production in oral mucosal wounds as compared with cutaneous wounds, which may contribute to decreased scar formation in mucosa.[3] Another isoform, TGF-β_3, which has antifibrotic properties, appears to be elevated in oral mucosal wounds as compared with skin wounds.[5]

Keratinocyte function is critical for effective wound reepithelialization for both mucosa and skin. It has been shown that equivalent-sized (1-mm) excisional wounds in oral mucosa completely reepithelialize in 24 hours versus only 25% in cutaneous wounds at 24 hours, suggesting a greater proliferative capacity in oral mucosal keratinocytes over skin keratinocytes. A study by Turabelidze and colleagues[2] also found that 13,710 genes are differentially expressed between the 2 tissues. This finding was unexpected, because the tissues share many histologic and functional characteristics, but it suggests that such dissimilarities may be critical to function. Turabelidze and colleagues[2] observed differential expression of specific proliferation and migration-associated genes in oral and skin epithelium. Several differentially expressed genes might influence keratinocyte migration and proliferation.[2]

One of the major differences between healing skin and mucosal wounds is the phenotypic differences in fibroblasts between the 2 tissues.[1] It

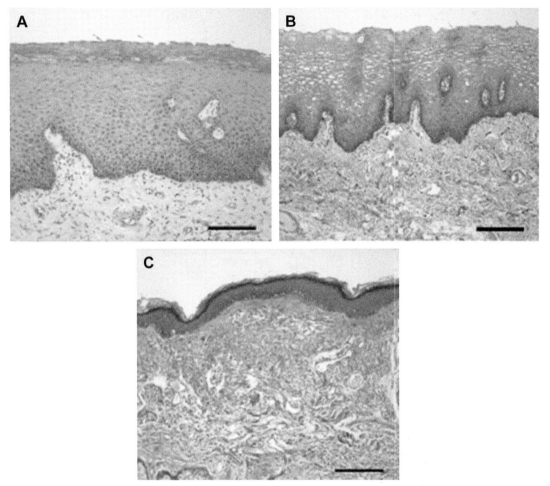

Fig. 2. Histologic comparison of keratinized mucosa (*A*), nonkeratinized mucosa (*B*), and skin (*C*). Scale bar = 200 μm (micrometers). (*From* Stephens P, Genève P. Non-epithelial oral mucosal progenitor cell populations. Oral Diseases 2007;13:1–10; with permission.)

may be these differences that make wound healing in mucosa so much faster and with less scarring than cutaneous wounds. In a study by Lee and Eun,[6] the proliferation, contraction, and synthesis of dermal and oral mucosal fibroblasts were compared. They found that oral mucosal fibroblasts proliferated more than dermal fibroblasts; however, the results were not significant. Dermal fibroblasts showed a significantly greater collagen gel contraction than oral mucosal fibroblasts. TGF-β_1 consistently increased the collagen gel contraction. Dermal fibroblasts had a greater response to TGF-β_1, which resulted in greater contraction. There were no significant differences in basal collagen synthesis between dermal and mucosal fibroblasts, however.[6] Some of the differences in wound healing and scar formation between skin and oral mucosa are probably due not only to differences in the responsiveness of fibroblasts to TGF-β_1 between

the tissues, but also the concentration of TGF-β_1 and other cytokines.

In a study using an animal model (red Duroc pig) by Mak and colleagues,[7] large oral mucosal wounds showed the following as compared with similar-sized skin wounds:

- Significantly reduced clinical scar formation and wound contraction
- Significantly better regeneration of connective tissue organization and reduced histologic scar formation
- Decreased number of macrophages
- Significantly fewer mast cells at 60 days after wounding
- Prolonged presence of increased number of myofibroblasts
- Lower density of blood vessels
- Lower numbers of TGF-β and pSmad3-positive connective tissue cells

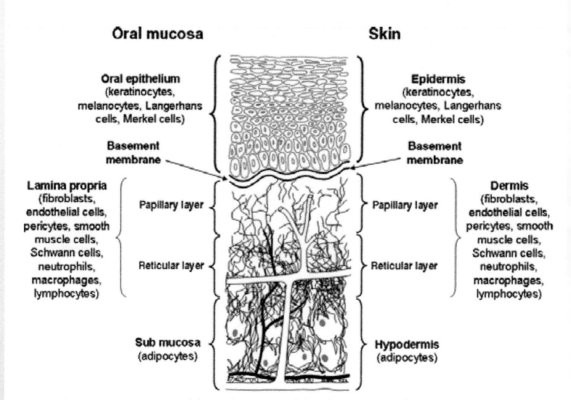

Fig. 3. Schematic representation of the oral mucosa and skin demonstrating the similarities in the epithelial, dermal, and subdermal layers. (*From* Stephens P, Genève P. Non-epithelial oral mucosal progenitor cell populations. Oral Diseases 2007;13:1–10; with permission.)

One surprising finding in this particular study was that mucosal wounds showed significantly greater numbers of myofibroblasts as compared with skin wounds. Typically, the prevention of wound contraction results in a less-overt scar, and higher myofibroblast numbers are reported to be associated with scarring. A study by Wong and colleagues[5] showed similar clinical and histologic scar assessment scores in human palatal mucosal wounds as compared with pig palatal mucosal wounds, suggesting that this animal model mimics human wound healing in the palatal mucosa.

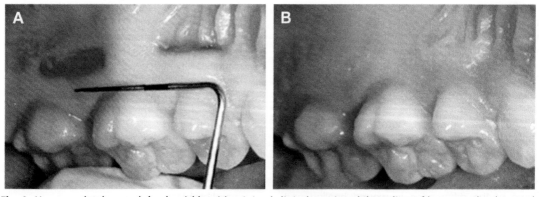

Fig. 4. Human palatal wounds heal quickly with minimal clinical scarring. (*A*) Healing of human palatal wounds (10 × 2 mm), 3 days (posterior) and 7 days (anterior) after wounding. (*B*) Healing of the same wounds after 60 days. (*From* Larjava H, Wiebe C, Gallant-Behm C, et al. Exploring scarless healing of oral soft tissues. J Can Dent Assoc 2011;77:B18; with permission.)

SCAR-PRODUCING DISEASE

A number of local or systemic diseases cause or mimic scarring of the mucosa. Without a history of traumatic or surgical injury to the affected tissue, a differential diagnosis is formulated based on history and physical examination findings. Some examples of diseases presenting as mucosal scarring include submucous fibrosis, basement membrane diseases (ie, pemphigus vulgaris and cicatricial pemphigoid), lichen planus, and proliferative verrucous leukoplakia to name a few examples.

Lichen Planus

Oral lichen planus is a common T-cell–mediated autoimmune disorder in which the resulting inflammation and keratinocyte proliferation results in a variable appearance. Typically, the lesions have the appearance of a leukoplakia; however, an erosive component may be seen (**Figs. 5–8**). There are reports of malignancy arising from these lesions. Skin lesions may develop in approximately 15% of cases.[8]

A variety of diseases, such as Stevens-Johnson syndrome and ocular cicatricial pemphigoid, may cause scars on the conjunctiva and secondary visual impairment. Due to similarities in tissue characteristics, autologous cultivated oral mucosal epithelial transplantation is a feasible treatment of scar phase of these severe ocular surface disorders.[9]

Submucous Fibrosis

One of the primary consequences of generalized mucosal scarring, wound contraction, is manifested in oral submucous fibrosis (OSF). OSF is a premalignant disorder associated with the

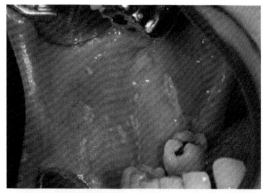

Fig. 6. Papular lichen planus. (*From* Scully C, Carrozzo M. Oral mucosal disease: lichen planus. Br J Oral Maxillofac Surg 2008;46:15–21; with permission.)

chewing of areca nut (betel nut), a habit that is prevalent in South Asian populations. The initial presentation of OSF is inflammation. Inflammation is followed by hypovascularity and fibrosis visible as blanching of the oral mucosa with a marblelike appearance. In the later advanced stage of OSF, a fibrous band that restricts mouth opening (trismus) is characteristic (**Fig. 9**). It causes further problems in oral hygiene, speech, mastication, and possibly swallowing. Development of fibrous bands in the lip leads to thickening and rubbery appearance.

The initial pathology of OSF is characterized by mixed inflammation and edema, and large fibroblasts. Later, collagen bundles with early hyalinization are seen, and the inflammatory infiltrate contains lymphocytes and plasma cells, occasionally resembling lichenoid mucositis.[10]

In more-advanced stages, OSF is characterized by formation of thick bands of collagen and hyalinization extending into the submucosal tissues and decreased vascularity (**Fig. 10**).

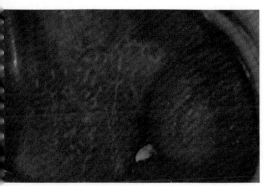

Fig. 5. Reticular lichen planus. (*From* Scully C, Carrozzo M. Oral mucosal disease: lichen planus. Br J Oral Maxillofac Surg 2008;46:15–21; with permission.)

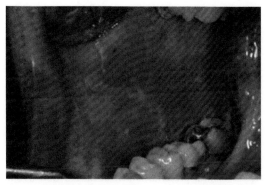

Fig. 7. Atrophic lichen planus. (*From* Scully C, Carrozzo M. Oral mucosal disease: lichen planus. Br J Oral Maxillofac Surg 2008;46:15–21; with permission.)

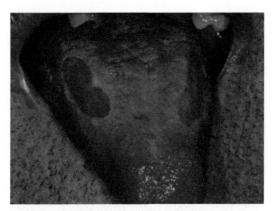

Fig. 8. Erosive lichen planus. (*From* Scully C, Carrozzo M. Oral mucosal disease: lichen planus. Br J Oral Maxillofac Surg 2008;46:15–21; with permission.)

Basement Membrane Diseases

Mucous membrane pemphigoid, also known as cicatricial pemphigoid, is a group of autoimmune blistering diseases that affects primarily the mucous membranes, namely the oral and conjunctival mucosa. Typically the disease follows a benign course with minimal residual scarring when it affects the oral mucosa only, but a more progressive course is usually encountered when the conjunctiva is affected.[11] Diagnosis requires direct immunofluorescence microscopy to demonstrate a linear deposition of immunoglobulin (Ig) G or IgA, or complement component 3 (C3), at the epithelial basement membrane (**Fig. 11**). Pemphigus vulgaris demonstrates acantholysis (loss of keratinocyte adhesion as a result

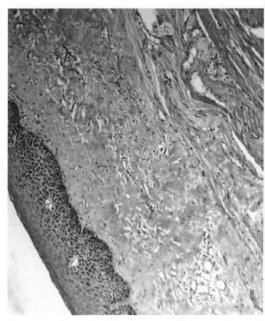

Fig. 10. Advanced OSF. (*From* Wollina U, Verma S, Fareedi M, et al. Oral submucous fibrosis: an update. Clin Cosmet Investig Dermatol 2015;8:193–204; with permission.)

of autoantibodies to intercellular adhesion molecules), which differs in that there is intraepithelial cleating rather than subepithelial clefting that is seen in cicatricial pemphigoid. Biopsies of these lesions should be taken from perilesional tissue (adjacent normal-appearing mucosa) and not

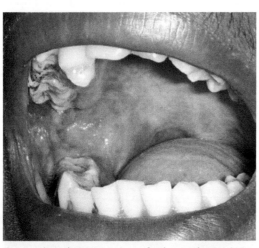

Fig. 9. Clinical presentation of advanced OSF. (*From* Wollina U, Verma S, Fareedi M, et al. Oral submucous fibrosis: an update. Clin Cosmet Investig Dermatol 2015;8:193–204; with permission.)

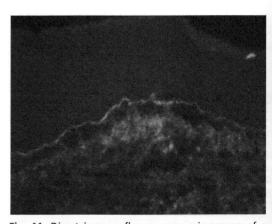

Fig. 11. Direct immunofluorescence microscopy of a biopsy specimen obtained from oral mucosa illustrates the linear deposit of C3 along the epithelial basement membrane in cicatricial pemphigoid. (*From* Chan LS. Ocular and oral mucous membrane pemphigoid (cicatricial pemphigoid). Clin Dermatol 2012;30:34–7; with permission.)

placed in formalin solution to perform direct immunofluorescence.

SCARS DUE TO INCISIONS/TRAUMA

Those of us who perform surgery on both the skin of the face and the oral, nasal, and conjunctival mucosa notice the rapid and relatively scarless healing of the mucosa compared with skin. Even so, incisions are still planned appropriately, care is taken during handling of the wound edges, and meticulous closure is performed so as to minimize scarring of the mucosal tissues as we would with skin. Certain areas of the oral mucosa tend to form scars due to webbing in the depth of the oral vestibule, however. This can be a problem particularly in the anterior mandible when approaching the chin for placement of a chin implant, osteotomy, or fracture repair. One method to avoid this problem is to place the incision away from the depth of the vestibule on the lip (**Fig. 12**). There are also anecdotal reports of intraoral vestibular incision closure using a running horizontal mattress suture rather than a typical running "baseball" suture to minimize scarring, presumably allowing for eversion of the wound edges (**Fig. 13**).

Chronic mucosal irritation is a common cause of mucosal scarring. These lesions frequently lead the clinician to rule out other possible causes when most times the offending irritant, such as a sharp dental restoration or prosthetic appliance, can be removed with resolution of the lesion. This is a common occurrence in traumatic ulcers, as seen in **Fig. 14**. Although an in-depth discussion of mucosal pathology is beyond the scope of this article, common abnormalities of the mucosa should be considered in one's differential diagnosis of mucosal scars.

BUCCAL MUCOSA HARVEST

Oral mucosa has been used as a donor tissue for reconstruction of various mucosal surfaces,

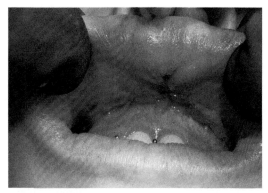

Fig. 13. Maxillary osteotomy incision closed using running horizontal mattress closure. Notice V-Y limb in the center to alleviate some flattening of the upper lip. (*Courtesy of* Erik Evans, DDS, MD, Cincinnati, OH.)

namely urethral, vaginal, pharyngeal, and conjunctival reconstruction due to its compatibility and similar characteristics to the recipient tissue.[12–15] The use of oral mucosa for urethral stricture reconstruction is commonplace. In a review of the literature regarding the use of oral mucosa in the reconstruction of urethral defects associated with urethral stricture and hypospadias/epispadias, there was an overall success rate of 76.4%.[13]

Özgenel and Özcan noted decreased contracture in vaginal construction for vaginal agenesis using buccal mucosa as compared with split-thickness skin grafts and no vaginal stenosis was encountered. The donor sites in this report healed uneventfully and with no change in mouth opening.[14,15] The buccal mucosa donor site may be closed primarily or left open to heal secondarily without an objectional scar.

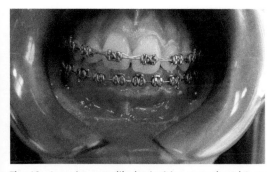

Fig. 12. Anterior mandibular incision scar placed 1 cm labial to depth of vestibule so as to avoid webbing. (*Courtesy of* Deepak Krishnan, DDS, Cincinnati, OH.)

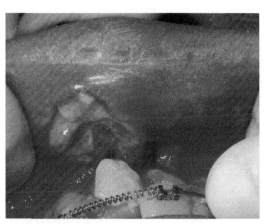

Fig. 14. Traumatic ulcer due to chronic mucosal irritation.

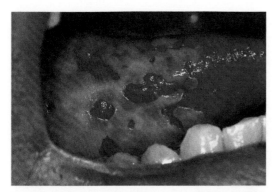

Fig. 15. Radiation-induced mucositis. (*From* Sciubba JJ, Goldenberg D. Oral complications of radiotherapy. Lancet Oncol 2006;7(2):175–83; with permission.)

EFFECTS OF RADIATION AND CHEMOTHERAPY

The treatment of malignancies of the head and neck frequently involve radiation therapy. Cells with rapid turnover, such as cancer cells, but also salivary gland and mucosal cells, are especially susceptible to the effects of radiation. These effects are greater in higher doses and with fields that involve the mucosal tissue and salivary glands. Direct radiation to the oral mucosa results in mucositis manifested as a loss of the surface epithelial layer with associated pain and burning that typically resolves after the cessation of radiation (**Fig. 15**).

The more problematic effects of radiation involve the necrosis of underlying bone, known as osteoradionecrosis (ORN), which causes dehiscence of the overlying mucosa. In some areas, oral mucosa directly overlies the periosteum of the

jaws. As a result of this unique anatomy and the presence of teeth, ORN and medication-related osteonecrosis (MRONJ) of the jaws may produce mucosal dehiscence and bony exposure. Although once thought only to be a result of the triad of hypoxia, hypocellularity, and hypovascularity, ORN is now believed to be a much more complex process.[16]

A similar clinical presentation to ORN, mucosal dehiscence secondary to underlying bony necrosis is seen in MRONJ. Typically a result of osteoclast-inhibiting medications used for bony metastases as well as lower doses used for osteoporosis, MRONJ is a relatively uncommon side effect of these medications (**Fig. 16**).

SUMMARY

Although by no means a comprehensive review of all possible causes of mucosal scarring and treatment, this article has touched on the structural and molecular basis for the "privileged" healing that takes place in mucosal tissues. Causes for mucosal scarring are described. There are many variables that contribute to scar formation during wound healing. Fortunately, mucous membranes, and specifically oral mucosa, heal rapidly and with minimal scar formation in comparison with skin. This is due to the privileged or "fetal" healing that takes place in mucosa due to a number of factors such as the activity of TGF-β isoforms, fibroblasts, and keratinocytes. There appear to be genetic, cellular-level differences between mucosal and cutaneous epithelium that afford the unique advantages in healing properties that are demonstrated by mucosa. The nonmobile anatomic locations around teeth make mucosal defects more difficult to manage in these locations; however, similar tissues taken from the palate may be grafted in these locations with good success.

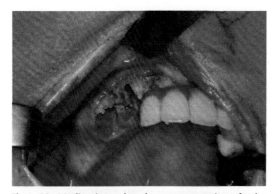

Fig. 16. Medication-related osteonecrosis of the maxilla. (*From* Assaf AT, Smeets R, Riecke B, et al. Incidence of bisphosphonate-related osteonecrosis of the jaw in consideration of primary diseases and concomitant therapies. Anticancer Res 2013;33(9):3917–24; with permission.)

REFERENCES

1. Enoch S, Wall I, Peake M, et al. Increased oral fibroblast lifespan is telomerase-independent. J Dent Res 2009;88(10):916–21.
2. Turabelidze A, Guo S, Chung AY, et al. Intrinsic differences between oral and skin keratinocytes. PLoS One 2014;9(9):e101480.
3. Schrementi ME, Ferreira AM, Zender C, et al. Site-specific production of TGF-β in oral mucosal and cutaneous wounds. Wound Repair Regen 2008;16:80–6.
4. Bussi M, De Stefani A, Milan F, et al. Is transposed skin transformed in major head and neck mucosal reconstruction? Acta Otolaryngol 1995;115:348–51.
5. Wong JW, Gallant-Behm C, Wiebe C, et al. Wound healing in oral mucosa results in reduced scar

formation as compared with skin: evidence from the red Duroc pig model and humans. Wound Repair Regen 2009;17:717–29.

6. Lee HG, Eun HC. Differences between fibroblasts cultured from oral mucosa and normal skin: implication to wound healing. J Dermatol Sci 1999;21:176–82.

7. Mak K, Manji A, Gallant-Behm C, et al. Scarless healing of oral mucosa is characterized by faster resolution of inflammation and control of myofibroblast action compared to skin wounds in the red Duroc pig model. J Dermatol Sci 2009;56:168–80.

8. Scully C, Carrozzo M. Oral mucosal disease: lichen planus. Br J Oral Maxillofac Surg 2008;46:15–21.

9. Nakamura T, Takea K, Inatomi T, et al. Long-term results of autologous cultivated oral mucosal epithelial transplantation in the scar phase of severe ocular surface disorders. Br J Ophthalmol 2011;95:942–6.

10. Wollina U, Verma S, Fareedi M, et al. Oral submucous fibrosis: an update. Clin Cosmet Investig Dermatol 2015;8:193–204.

11. Chan LS. Ocular and oral mucous membrane pemphigoid (cicatricial pemphigoid). Clin Dermatol 2012;30:34–7.

12. Eppley BL. A simplified technique for harvesting large buccal mucosal grafts. J Oral Maxillofac Surg 1997;55:891–2.

13. Markiewicz MR, Lukose MA, Margarone JE, et al. The oral mucosa graft: a systematic review. J Urol 2007;178:387–94.

14. Özgenel Y, Özcan M. Neovaginal construction with buccal mucosa grafts. Plast Reconstr Surg 2003; 111:2250–4.

15. Shah SB, Tauro DP. Clinical and histological basis for the use of nasolabial tissues in the surgical management of oral submucous fibrosis. J Oral Maxillofac Surg 2015;73:2251.e1-12.

16. Lyons A, Osher J, Warner E, et al. Osteoradionecrosis: a review of current concepts in defining the extent of the disease and a new classification proposal. Br J Oral Maxillofac Surg 2014;52:392–5.

Treating Scars to the Neck

Richard D. Gentile, MD, MBA

KEYWORDS

- Scar • Neck • Morbidity • Face

KEY POINTS

- Scarring of the neck is a common complication of burns, surgeries, physical disorders/disease, and traumatic injuries, affecting millions of people every year.
- Scarring of the neck can be accompanied by additional morbidities caused by the limitation of functional motion of the neck by severe scarring, is the neck being more dynamic than the face.
- Many treatment options and modalities have been used for reduction and prevention of scar formation, including topical steroids, intralesional steroids, interferon, 5-fluorouracil, silicone gel, radiation, laser therapy, and surgeries.
- The most important aspect of patient care with regard to treating scars of the neck is that patients should have realistic expectations of the most likely outcome of the treatment; that is, that the visibility and problems associated with the scar will be lessened by the treatment but that the treatment is unlikely to result in elimination of the neck scar.

INTRODUCTION

Scarring of the face and neck are of great concern to patients because of their high visibility and the distortion of facial and neck features that become socially important in the overall appearance of the patient. The goal of any surgeon in the revision of neck scars should be improvement to the point of optimal camouflage,[1] and it should be noted that eliminating neck scars is highly unlikely. Unlike facial scars, the neck has a dynamic component in the motion of the face and neck, and correction of neck scars may be necessary to restore normal function of head and neck rotation; specifically, flexion, extension, and rotation. Patients presenting with neck scars or scar concerns in general should be advised that realistic expectations are necessary to establish a rapport with the patient in order to achieve a successful end point in the treatment. Discussion of neck scar treatment should emphasize that the treatment is to lessen the adverse effects that scarring

has produced and that no treatment is capable of eliminating the scar.

CAUSES OF NECK SCARRING AND SCAR FORMATION

Neck scarring can occur as a result of trauma, burns, physical disorders/disease, or surgical intervention, either elective or emergent. Normal scar formation after ordinary wound repair usually results in acceptable postoperative appearance of neck scars. Unsatisfactory neck scarring can result from extensive tissue loss or damage, complications or infections of the wound, or poor technique in wound closure. Poor wound healing can also result from concurrent illness, poor nutrition, and immunosuppression. Abnormal wound healing, hypertrophic scarring, and keloid formation can also result as consequences of the wound healing process. Common surgical scars that may heal unfavorably include those for carotid surgery, thyroid surgery, tracheotomy,

Gentile Facial Plastic & Aesthetic Laser Center, 821 Kentwood Suite C, Boardman, OH 44512, USA
E-mail address: dr-gentile@msn.com

Facial Plast Surg Clin N Am 25 (2017) 99–104
http://dx.doi.org/10.1016/j.fsc.2016.08.009
1064-7406/17/© 2016 Elsevier Inc. All rights reserved.

submandibular gland removal, or other more extensive head and neck surgery procedures.

CHARACTERIZATION OF UNFAVORABLE NECK SCARS

An ideal scar is thin and flat, has a good color match with the surrounding skin, is oriented along the relaxed skin tension lines (RSTLs), and does not produce any distortion of adjacent tissues.[2] A scar may impede function, as in the case of a contracture or limitation of motion. A scar may cause discomfort, tightness, or even pain. Frequently scars cause cosmetic deformity and patients may seek treatment merely to look more normal. Scars are often associated with an unpleasant memory or reminders of a traumatic past, and the patient may seek to erase the memories by erasing the scar. The causes of unsatisfactory neck scarring are similar to those of scars of the facial area, and can be directly related to the location of the wound, cause of the wound, and degree of tissue loss. Wounds that occur in areas of increased tension, like those overlying the mandible or those that are perpendicular to the resting skin tension lines, may heal with unfavorable consequences, particularly with increased width. Wounds with a large degree of soft tissue injury, such as avulsion injuries, deep thermal wounds, or gunshot wounds, and severe abrasions with epidermal or dermal loss, may also result in unfavorable scars. Unfavorable scars may be wide, have irregular contours, or be hypertrophied or retracted with uneven tissue contours. Uneven closure of surgical or traumatic wounds caused by poor layered approximation can also contribute to uneven contours with step-offs or distortion in which straight lines along the edge of a wound bulge toward the center, also known as a pincushion deformity. A version of the pincushion deformity is the trapdoor deformity.

TOPICAL AND INJECTABLE TREATMENT OF NECK SCARRING

Intralesional corticosteroids are a frequently used adjunctive treatment of hypertrophic scars and keloids. Their mechanism of action involves reduction of fibroblast proliferation and collagen synthesis as well as suppressing inflammatory mediators.[3] In addition, triamcinolone acetonide seems to cause a sizable decrease in antitrypsin and macroglobulin levels, both of which are increased in keloids and are inhibitors of collagenase.[4] Fluorouracil, a pyrimidine analogue with antimetabolite activity, has been used extensively in the treatment of cancer and as an adjunct to glaucoma surgery. More recently, it has been shown to have some efficacy in the treatment of hypertrophic scars and keloids. Fluorouracil has been shown to target rapidly proliferating fibroblasts in dermal wounds, thus inhibiting excessive collagen production.[5] More specifically, fluorouracil blocks the transforming growth factor beta (TGF-β)-2 gene in human fibroblasts, a known proinflammatory cytokine present in adult wounds that scar.[6] Imiquimod cream, 5%, is a topical immune response modifier that stimulates interferon, a proinflammatory cytokine that increases collagen breakdown. It has also been shown to enhance the local production of tumor necrosis factors and interleukins.[7] Bleomycin is a cytotoxic antibiotic isolated from a *Streptomyces verticillus* strain commonly used in the treatment of certain neoplasms as well as recalcitrant warts in dermatology. It acts by binding to both double-stranded and single-stranded DNA, leading to breaks in the structure. On histology, bleomycin has been shown to cause necrosis of keratinocytes and induces the expression of several adhesion molecules.[8] Silicone gel is a cross-linked polymer of dimethyl siloxane used as an impregnated elastic sheet, silicone gel sheeting (SGS), silicone cream, or a topical gel. It is noninvasive and has the advantages of being inexpensive, painless, and easy to use. The exact mechanism by which SGS exerts its effects remains unclear and continues to be a subject of controversy. Some investigators have suggested that it is the hydration of the stratum corneum rather than the inherent properties of the silicone that affects wound healing.[9,10] In 2004, Hanasono and colleagues[11] performed in vitro testing on human fibroblasts from various tissues, including normal, keloid, and fetal skin. Their results suggested that silicone gel is responsible for increased basic fibroblast growth factor levels in normal and fetal dermal fibroblasts and acts as a modulator in the expression of such growth factors.[11]

LASER AND RADIOFREQUENCY THERAPY FOR NECK SCARRING

Lasers were first used in the treatment of scars in 1978. Laser scar treatment can be performed with a multitude of devices and the energy-based devices are divided into the following 3 categories: ablative, nonablative, and fractional technologies (ablative and nonablative). The 3 types differ in their method and extent of thermal damage, length of downtime, adverse effect profiles, and degrees of efficacy. The first laser used to treat hypertrophic scars and keloids was the continuous wave argon.[12] Despite encouraging early reports, subsequent studies showed limited efficacy and high incidence of side effects.[13] Then, the neodymium:yttrium-aluminum-garnet (1064 nm) laser and continuous wave CO_2 laser (10,600 nm) were described in the early 1980s as alternatives to argon by selectively inhibiting collagen production.[14] However, results showed failure to inhibit keloid formation and recurrence of lesions 1 year after treatment.[15] The theory of selective photothermolysis, which was introduced in the early 1980s, has resulted in the invention of pulsed lasers that provide target selectivity, reducing the thermal damage and scarring.[16] The lasers delivering the most improvement over the years are the pulsed dye lasers and fractionated lasers. Fractionated CO_2 laser seems to be an encouraging approach in treatment of keloids. The CO_2 laser decreases fibroblasts proliferation, increases basic fibroblast growth factor production (ie, reduces collagen synthesis), and inhibits TGF-β1 secretion (ie, increases collagen synthesis).[17] Fractionated resurfacing may improve hypertrophic scars through vaporization or coagulation of microscopic dermal columns and this in turn stimulates collagen production and remodeling.[18] Pulsed dye laser affects blood vessels of keloids and hypertrophic scars through the concept of selective photothermolysis, in which the light energy emitted from pulsed dye laser is absorbed by hemoglobin, generating heat and leading to coagulation necrosis.[19] Vascular changes were also noted in pulsed dye laser–irradiated tissue, beginning with occlusion of the papillary vascular plexus and evolving to longitudinal rearrangement of blood vessels and cross-filling between vessels of adjacent territories.[20] A new option for neck scar treatment is fractional microneedle radiofrequency devices. The 32-gauge or 34-gauge insulated bipolar microneedles help to remodel scars by softening and then performing small ablations of the scar tissue, which can be replace by a less fibrous matrix. The fractionation of these devices is similar to the fractionated lasers.

TREATMENT OF NECK SCARRING: SURGICAL

The surgical treatment of neck scars can be grouped into 4 major categories. The first of these, and the most commonly used, are excisional techniques. Of the excisional techniques, the most common are fusiform excisions. Fusiform excisions are useful for small scars that are wide or depressed and lie close to the RSTLs. Fusiform excision also works well with neck scars that are hypertrophic. Classically, the angle at the end of the excision needs to be less than 30°. In patients with small raised scars, a shave excision may be useful in reducing the visibility of the neck scar.

Serial excision as a method of scar revision is done in stages, which places less tension on the incision line than if a greater excision was performed. Serial excision relies on skin distensibility over time with smaller sequential excision. Serial excision can be used to move a scar to a better location. In patients with large areas of tissue loss from trauma or burns, serial excision is useful to sequentially remove abnormal-appearing grafted areas. Tissue expansion can be used in conjunction with serial incision. The second class of scar revision techniques involves the alteration of scar polarity or irregularizing the scar by breaking up large straight-line scars in order to reposition the scar to better align with RSTLs. These techniques also help to alleviate webs or clefts, reposition facial landmarks, or provide elongation to an unbalanced scar. The techniques are well known and include Z-plasty, W-plasty, and geometric broken-line closure. Z-plasty is commonly used for scar elongation, releasing of scar contractures, or to change the direction of the scar (from perpendicular to parallel to RSTLs.) Z-plasty can also be used to change a displaced anatomic point, raising or lowering it. W-plasty is performed by excising consecutive small triangles on each side of a wound and imbricating the resultant triangular flaps. Unlike Z-plasty, W-plasty does not cause overall lengthening of the scar. Geometric broken-line closure is a series of random, irregular, geometric shapes cut from one side of a wound and interdigitated with the mirror image of this pattern on the opposite side. All shapes should be between 5 and 7 mm in any dimension for improved camouflage. Geometric broken-line closure does not affect the length of the scar.

Abrasion techniques are used as a primary method of scar correction and also after surgical correction of unfavorable scars. Abrasion techniques are not as commonly used on the neck as on the face because of the reduced thickness of the neck skin with fewer dermoepithelial units available for reepithelialization during wound healing. Dermabrasion is usually performed with motorized or gas-driven devices with attached wire brushes or diamond fraises. Extreme care must be taken with dermabrasion not to burrow too deeply past the papillary dermis or additional scarring may result. The reduced thickness of neck skin makes this a delicate procedure and one that should be performed with extreme care. Dermabrasion can be performed to enhance the results of other scar revision techniques, such as Z-plasty, W-plasty, and geometric broken-line closure.

Skin and soft tissue grafts and flaps make up the final category of neck scar revision options. Because of the flexibility of neck skin, primary

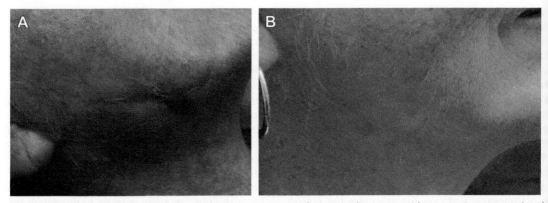

Fig. 1. Patient is shown before and after undergoing injections of triamcinolone acetonide suspension 40 mg/ml and staged polychromatic light treatments with intense pulsed light as well as fractionated ablative carbon dioxide laser.

closure is possible in many excisional techniques and partial-thickness or full-thickness skin grafting is not commonly used except in procedures in which very large defects are produced. Likewise, advancement, rotation, transposition, and interposition flaps, and rarely free flaps, are necessary for neck scar revision unless severe functional morbidity exists because of large defects with severe contracture.

ANCILLARY AND OTHER TREATMENTS OF NECK SCARRING

Pressure therapy has been a common form of conservative management in the treatment of scars since the late 1960s.[21] Several mechanisms have been proposed to explain how pressure therapy exerts its effect on hypertrophic scars. Pressure therapy is thought to accelerate wound maturation by thinning of the dermis, decreasing edema, and decreasing blood flow and oxygen to create a hypoxic environment. This hypoxic environment results in fibroblast degeneration and decreased collagen synthesis.[22] Radiotherapy has been used for the treatment of keloids. Its use as a monotherapy has been shown to be inadequate for the treatment of keloids,[23] which is why it is frequently combined with surgical resection. The suggested mechanism of action of radiation is the control of collagen synthesis by affecting fibroblast proliferation and inducing apoptosis.[24]

CASE STUDIES

The patient is a 62-year-old woman with trauma to the lower face and upper neck. After primary wound closure done under emergency conditions the patient was left with an irregular scar that was hypertrophic in some areas (**Fig. 1**A). The patient underwent injections of triamcinolone acetonide

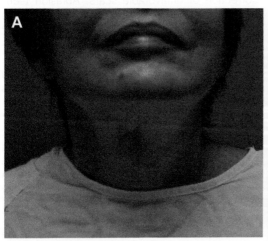
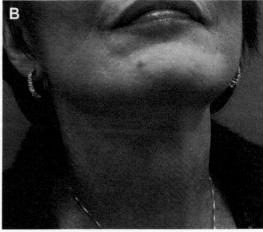

Fig. 2. A 61-year-old woman with neck trauma. (*A*) Depressed neck scar with irregular contours. (*B*) After surgery, showing a more evenly contoured neck with less noticeable scar tissue and contour irregularity.

suspension 40 mg/mL and staged polychromatic light treatments with intense pulsed light as well as fractionated ablative CO_2 laser. Her posttreatment photographs show improvement in color, texture, contour, and magnitude of scar tissue (**Fig. 1**B).

The patient is a 61-year-old woman with neck trauma who shows a depressed neck scar with irregular contours (**Fig. 2**A). She was treated with scar revision that included soft tissue rearrangement and her postoperative photographs show a more evenly contoured neck with much less noticeable scar tissue and contour irregularity (**Fig. 2**B).

SUMMARY

Scarring of the neck is a common complication of burns, surgeries, physical disorders/disease, and traumatic injuries affecting millions of people every year. The appearance of neck scarring can be disturbing to patients both physically and psychologically. Scarring of the neck can be accompanied by additional morbidities because of the limitation of functional motion of the neck by severe scarring, the neck being more dynamic than the face. Many treatment options and modalities have been used for reduction and prevention of scar formation, including topical steroids, intralesional steroids, interferon, 5-fluorouracil, silicone gel, radiation, laser therapy, and surgeries. There is no general consensus in the literature as to the optimal treatment of neck scarring. The most important aspect of patient care with regard to treating scars of the neck is that patients should have realistic expectations of the most likely outcome of the treatment; that is, that the visibility and problems associated with the scar will be lessened by the treatment but that the treatment is unlikely to result in elimination of the neck scar.

REFERENCES

1. Thomas JR, Ehlert TK. Scar revision. In: Papel ID, Nachlas NE, editors. Facial plastic and reconstructive surgery. St Louis (MO): Mosby; 1992. p. 45–55.
2. Sharma M, Wakure A. Scar Revision. Indian J Plast Surg 2013;46(2):408–18.
3. Katz BE. Silicone gel sheeting in scar therapy. Cutis 1995;56(1):65–7.
4. Diegelmann RF, Bryant CP, Cohen IK. Tissue alpha-globulins in keloid formation. Plast Reconstr Surg 1977;59(3):418–23.
5. Chen MA, Davidson TM. Scar management: prevention and treatment strategies. Curr Opin Otolaryngol Head Neck Surg 2005;13(4):242–7.
6. Wendling J, Marchand A, Mauviel A, et al. 5-Fluorouracil blocks transforming growth factor-beta-induced alpha 2 type I collagen gene (COL1A2) expression in human fibroblasts via c-Jun NH2-terminal kinase/activator protein-1 activation. Mol Pharmacol 2003;64(3):707–13.
7. Miller RL, Gerster JF, Owens ML, et al. Imiquimod applied topically: a novel immune response modifier and new class of drug. Int J Immunopharmacol 1999;21(1):1–14.
8. Templeton SF, Solomon AR, Swerlick RA. Intradermal bleomycin injections into normal human skin: a histopathologic and immunopathologic study. Arch Dermatol 1994;130(5):577–83.
9. Chang CC, Kuo YF, Chiu HC, et al. Hydration, not silicone, modulates the effects of keratinocytes on fibroblasts. J Surg Res 1995;59(6):705–11.
10. Suetak T, Sasai S, Zhen YX, et al. Effects of silicone gel sheet on the stratum corneum hydration. Br J Plast Surg 2000;53(6):503–7.
11. Hanasono MM, Lum J, Carroll LA, et al. The effect of silicone gel on basic fibroblast growth factor levels in fibroblast cell culture. Arch Facial Plast Surg 2004;6(2):88–93.
12. Ginsbach G, Kohnel W. The treatment of hypertrophic scars and keloids by argon laser: clinical data and morphological findings. Plast Surg Forum 1978;1:61–7.
13. Hulsbergen HJP, Roskam Y, van Gemert MJ. Treatment of keloids and hypertrophic scars with an argon laser. Lasers Surg Med 1986;6(1):72–5.
14. Aberge RP, Dwyer RM, Meeker CA, et al. Laser treatment of keloids: a clinical trial and in vitro study with Nd:YAG laser. Lasers Surg Med 1984;4(3):291–5.
15. Lim TC, Tan WT. Carbon dioxide laser for keloids. Plast Reconstr Surg 1991;88(6):1111.
16. Anderson RR, Parrish JA. Selective photothermolysis: precise microsurgery by selective absorption of pulsed radiation. Science 1983;220(4596):524–7.
17. Scrimali L, Lomeo G, Tamburino S, et al. Laser CO_2 versus radiotherapy in treatment of keloid scars. J Cosmet Laser Ther 2012;14:94–7.
18. Hultman CS, Edkins RE, Lee CN, et al. Shine on: review of laser- and light-based therapies for the treatment of burn scars. Dermatol Res Pract 2012;2012: 243651.
19. Liu A, Moy RL, Ross EV, et al. Pulsed dye laser and pulsed dye laser–mediated photodynamic therapy in the treatment of dermatologic disorders. Dermatol Surg 2012;38(3):351–66.
20. Lack EB, Rachel JD. Resolution of retracted scar after 585-nm pulse dye laser surgery. J Cosmet Laser Ther 2004;6:149–51.
21. Linares HA, Larson DL, Willis-Galstaun BA. Historical notes on the use of pressure in the treatment of hypertrophic scars or keloids. Burns 1993;19(1): 17–21.

22. Jensen LL, Parshley PF. Postburn scar contractures: histology and effects of pressure treatment. J Burn Care Res 1984;5(2):119–23.

23. Borok TL, Bray M, Sinclair I, et al. Role of ionizing irradiation for 393 keloids. Int J Radiat Oncol Biol Phys 1988;15(4):865870.

24. Ogawa R, Mitsuhashi K, Hyakusoku H, et al. Postoperative electron beam irradiation therapy for keloids and hypertrophic scars: retrospective study of 147 cases followed for more than 18 months. Plast Reconstr Surg 2003;111(2):547–55.

Contemporary Topics Relevant to Facial Scarring

Laser-Assisted Delivery to Treat Facial Scars

Jill S. Waibel, MD[a,b,c,*], Ashley Rudnick, BS[d]

KEYWORDS

- Laser assisted drug delivery • Ablative fractional laser • Facial scars

KEY POINTS

- The treatment of disfiguring facial scars has been reinvigorated with recent advances in technology.
- Laser-assisted drug delivery (LAD) is an emerging technology to achieve greater penetration by existing topical medications and drugs to reach desired targets in the skin.
- LADs allows us to alter the stratum corneum, epidermis and/or dermis to facilitate increased penetration of a drug or device to a specific target.
- This emerging concept is bridging medicine with technology; however, the drugs have not been formulated for this type of delivery and so this science is "off-label."

INTRODUCTION

Facial Scars

There are few medical situations as distressing as that of a child or adult whose life has been permanently altered by tragedy. The profound physical, mental, financial, and psychological damage brought on by such calamitous events often are accompanied by significant scarring. When the scarring is on the face, patients have severe physical and psychological stress. The treatment of facial scars is a multispecialty endeavor for optimal patient recovery.

Current Treatments

Scar rehabilitation is the restoring of form and function in scar patients. There are multiple therapeutic approaches have been used in scar management, including surgery (z-plasty), physical therapy, compression, silicone sheeting, corticosteroid therapy, and laser therapy. Leading the

way in scar treatments are lasers, which are a scientifically precise and effective treatment modalities to rehabilitate and improve scars. Laser has added a powerful tool to improve scar symptoms and deformities. Given the established benefit of lasers with scars[1,2] new methods to synergistically improve scars are being studied. At the forefront is laser-assisted delivery (LAD) of drugs, molecules and cells for scar rehabilitation. LAD is a new delivery system (vs oral, intravenous) that enables physician to uniformly distribute drug, cell, or cosmeceutical in microscopic channels to desired depth in cutaneous tissue. Without exception thus far, ablative fractional laser has been found to enhance the local uptake of any drug or substance applied to the skin through any fractional ablative tunnels can be used for LAD systems of a variety of drugs, topical agents, and other living tissue. These zones may be used immediately postoperatively to deliver drugs and other substances to synergistically create an

Disclosure Statement: J.S. Waibel, disclose the following "relevant financial relationship(s)" with commercial or financial conflicts of interest and any funding sources. Serve as a consultant: MiraDry, Lumenis, Sciton. Speaking Honoraria: Lumenis, Sciton, Syneron/Candela. Research Grant: Galderma, Lumenis, Lutronics, Sciton, Syneron/Candela.
[a] Private Practice: Miami Dermatology and Laser Institute, 7800 Southwest 87th Avenue, Suite B200, Miami, FL 33173, USA; [b] Baptist Hospital, Miami, FL, USA; [c] Dermatology Faculty, Miller School of Medicine, University of Miami, Miami, FL, USA; [d] 7800 Southwest 87th Avenue, Suite B200, Miami, FL 33173, USA
* Corresponding author. 7800 Southwest 87th Avenue, Suite B200, Miami, FL 33173.
E-mail address: jwaibelmd@miamidermlaser.com

Facial Plast Surg Clin N Am 25 (2017) 105–117
http://dx.doi.org/10.1016/j.fsc.2016.08.010
1064-7406/17/Published by Elsevier Inc.

enhanced scar therapeutic response to drug or substance applied to the skin.

History of Laser-Assisted Delivery

Topical drug delivery is essential in the treatment of many cutaneous conditions. The efficacy of topical therapy depends on the penetration of viable skin. However, therapeutic benefit is ultimately limited by absorption of the medication through the skin's inherent barrier properties. The stratum corneum, the outermost layer of the skin, serves as the rate-limiting step for percutaneous penetration and only 1% to 5% of topically applied drugs absorb into the skin.[3]

Drugs that are semilipophilic (uncharged/nonpolar) and small (<500 Da) may pass through the stratum corneum because the corneocytes are embedded in a lipid matrix. Drugs that are lipophilic and large hydrophilic drugs are not suited for delivery through intact skin. Furthermore, many medications are too large to penetrate and currently require either an injectable or systemic delivery.

Strategies to enhance topical drug delivery include chemical (solvents, surfactants), biochemical (nanoparticle, lipid synthesis inhibitors), and physical methods (tape stripping, sonophoresis, microneedling). The most commonly used in today's topical drug world is chemical modifications. These approaches are used to remove or alter the stratum corneum and have had variable success with improving drug delivery.

When a drug enters the skin and remains within the skin it is called *penetration*; this is how most dermatology drug targets within the skin and function to improve disease. *Transdermal delivery* and absorption means a drug has crossed the skin barrier and entered the bloodstream.[3] Transdermal patches have been used since the 1970s, but are limited to drugs with a low molecular mass (<500 Da) and high lipophilicity.[3–5]

Laser-assisted drug delivery
Laser-assisted drug delivery is an evolving modality first published in 2002,[6] which may allow for a greater precision of depth penetration by existing topical medications and more efficient transcutaneous delivery of drug molecules. Fractional ablative lasers, either carbon dioxide (CO_2) or erbium:YAG (Er:YAG), provide a novel way to create a conduit in the stratum corneum, epidermal, and dermal layers in a predictable and controlled pattern resulting in the potential for increased penetration of topically applied molecules. Both CO_2 and Er:YAG are infrared lasers that heat skin tissue to greater than 100°C and cause vaporization. The Er:YAG has an absorption

coefficient of 2×10^7/cm and owing to high absorption of water it takes less energy to ablate tissue. The CO_2 has an absorption coefficient 2×10^6 $cm^{-1}\ m^{-1}$ and takes higher energies to ablate tissue resulting in increased thermal damage compared with the Er:YAG laser.

Ablative fractional resurfacing creates vertical channels of ablation surrounded by thin layers of coagulated tissue known as microthermal zones (MTZ).[5] The creation of these channels theoretically serves as access points for drug delivery and allow for transport of actives deeper into the skin.

LAD is a more efficient transcutaneous delivery of large drug molecules, and potentially a way of delivering systemic medication via a transcutaneous route.[3] Topical drug delivery has many advantages over traditional oral medication. With dermatologic disease, topical administration of therapies directly to the skin limit systemic toxicity. In addition, drug degradation by the gastrointestinal system and first-pass liver metabolism can be avoided with laser cutaneous delivery.

The goals for a cutaneous delivery system include increasing the ability to attain a therapeutic target, decreasing amount of drug needed to deliver, decreasing adverse events to other organs and ease of use for patients. LAD is a new emerging concept bridging medicine with technology to improve health care.

Clinical Applications of Laser-Assisted Delivery

Various dermatologic conditions have been studied with LAD including dysplasia, nonmelanoma skin cancer, psoriasis, inflammatory conditions, local anesthesia, and scars. Studies of LAD have shown without exception that ablative fractional laser pretreatment has been found to enhance the local uptake of any drug or substance applied to the skin.

Investigated dermatologic drugs included lidocaine, 5-aminolevulinic acid (ALA), methyl-5-amnolevulinate (MAL), 5-fluorouracil (5-FU), ascorbic acid, diclofenac, ingenol mebutate, imiquimod, methotrexate, and vaccinations.[7–18] Specifically in the arena of LAD of scars, compounds studied include corticosteroids, ascorbic acid, 5-FU, platelet-rich plasma, and stem cells.[8,19–21]

Which Laser Is the Best Laser-Assisted Delivery?

Haedersdal and colleagues[22] studied a variety of physical techniques that disturbed the stratum corneum to study which modality best enhanced protoporphyrin IX accumulation. Modalities studied included nonablative fractional laser, ablative fractional laser, microneedling, microdermabrasion, curettage, and control. Of all these modalities only ablative laser therapy has the ability to destroy the stratum corneum, epidermal and dermal layers of skin in a predictable and controlled manner, resulting in the potential for increased penetration of topically applied molecules. This study showed the fractional ablative laser was superior enhancing protoporphyrin IX accumulation in the dermis versus the other modalities.

Nonablative lasers do disrupt the dermal epidermal junction, but do not create an opening for larger molecules to gain access to the dermis. This is best understood by histologic differences between nonablative fractional lasers and ablative fractional lasers (**Fig. 1**).

Laser Dosimetry for Laser-Assisted Delivery

To understand how to best treat facial scars with a LAD system specifically requires an understanding of basic LAD dosimetry strategies. By calibrating laser settings, it is possible to influence drug amount delivered, drug delivery rate, and drug biodistribution. Ablative fractional lasers may be tailored by laser settings including channel density, depth of the channels, as well as the coagulation around the ablated channel to increase drug deposition into targeted cutaneous levels.

Channel Density and Laser-Assisted Delivery

The definition of channel density is the ablated skin surface area. This density can be adjusted via laser spot size or the number of applied channels in a fixed scan pattern. The effect of channel density on rate and extent of drug delivery has been studied for lidocaine[18] and MAL.[23] Bachhav and colleagues[23] studied the effect of channel density on permeation of topical lidocaine in an in vitro porcine model using Er:YAG fractional ablative laser. Their initial hypothesis was that increasing the number of laser channels would increase the overall drug delivery. Channel densities studied included 0 (control), 150, 300, 450, and 900 channels per 3 cm^2 with a fixed laser fluence at 24 hours. There was no difference in cumulative permeation between 450 and 900 channels at 6 hours or 300, 450, and 900 pores at 24 hours. Increased permeation of lidocaine occurred with increasing channels up to 450. The authors concluded there is a minimum channel density to achieve maximum increase in drug penetration but that increasing channel density beyond this will not improve permeation. In both literature and experience, there seems to be a plateau around 100 channels/cm^2. Low density is favored in LAD of drugs. Increasing density may increase the possibility of systemic absorption of that drug.

Laser Channel Depth Effect on Laser-Assisted Delivery

Laser depth describes the depth of the laser channels and can be adjusted by pulse energy. Higher pulse energies in fractional ablative laser give deeper ablated laser channels. Deeper channels were initially expected to induce a greater dermal uptake of drug; however, inconsistent data on

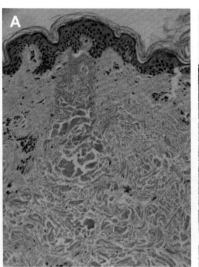
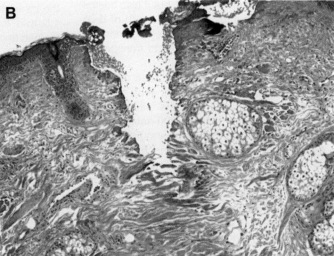

Fig. 1. (*A*) Histology of nonablative laser showing heated collagen but no open ablative channels. (*B*) Histology of Erbium:YAG ablative laser showing open channels creating a doorway for topical penetration of drugs, cells, and cosmeceuticals.

the influence of laser channel depths have been published.[23]

Early studies with lidocaine studied the effect of channel depth on rate and extent of drug delivery. Bachhav and colleagues[23] used an in vitro porcine model with Er:YAG laser with increasing laser fluences from 150 to 200 microns. The greater fluence resulted in greater channel depth. Lower fluences in some cases resulted in removal of stratum corneum without going deeper into the epidermis and higher fluences showed channels through the epidermis and dermis, thus supporting the notion that the laser is tunable to the desired depth but probably needs to be closer to 200 microns to reach the dermis. However, this study was performed in porcine in vitro model not human. Also in this study it was noted that greater fluence did not result in statistically significantly greater cumulative lidocaine permeation with fixed channel numbers. In addition, changing the fluence did not result in greater total lidocaine deposition. The authors concluded that lidocaine delivery is enhanced with LAD, but the transport was independent of fluence, suggesting that even low fluences are sufficient to enhance lidocaine delivery.

In a well-performed porcine LAD study, Oni and colleagues[18] hypothesized that a greater channel depth would lead to greater transdermal absorption. This experiment tested fractional ablative channels at 25, 50, 250, and 500 microns. The result of this study revealed maximum absorption occurred at 250 micron depth. Oni and colleagues concluded this may be owing to vascular plexus between 100 to 300 microns in porcine skin.

Additional research is needed, but it also seems that the drug properties affect the depth of drug delivered, depending on both how charge and hydrophobic versus hydrophilic affects transport in channels.

The optimal depth for scars most likely relates to the thickness of the scar. Scars tend to have abnormal collagen, mainly in the papillary and reticular dermis, lying between 200 and 2000 microns in depth. When treating scars, the authors recommend trying to establish and treat the full depth of the scar. Another study by Sakamoto and colleagues[24] showed no difference in drug penetration for either low channel densities or high channel densities. An in vivo porcine model with CO_2 fractional ablative laser using 100, 200, and 400 MTZ/cm^2 densities for ALA in photodynamic therapy revealed increasing density did not enhance ALA delivery to deeper skin layers, and this may be unique to the chemical properties of ALA.

Coagulation Zone in Laser-Assisted Delivery

The coagulation zone in fractional ablative laser treatment is defined by the thickness of coagulated tissue surrounding the ablative zone. This may be adjusted with some laser systems by the total energy delivered and turning on or off coagulation. The diffusion coefficient of coagulated tissue is less than normal tissue; thus, ablative zones with coagulated tissue have a lower diffusivity. This may have an effect on drug delivery in that a thick coagulation zone may serve as a secondary diffusion barrier and create a drug reservoir in these channels, which we may find to be a positive attribute if we are aiming to delivery drug to the dermis, and do not want systemic delivery. Conversely, no coagulation zone may be better for systemic delivery goals.

Molecular Weight and Drug Diffusion in Laser-Assisted Delivery

An investigation by Haak and colleagues[25] evaluated laser density and molecular weight of polyethylene glycols of increasing molecular weights from 250 to 4000 Da. The polyethylene glycols were applied to the skin after fractional ablative CO_2 laser at densities of 25, 100, 225, and 440 MTZ/cm^2. Mass spectrometry and nuclear magnetic resonance spectroscopy revealed greater densities resulted in greater transdermal delivery although no statistically significant differences of greater than 100 MTZ/cm^2. Uptake of the lowest molecular weight was favored. Haedersdal and colleagues[26] studied in vivo LAD of MAL in a porcine model with a CO_2 fractional ablative laser. The experiment studied diffusion distances from the laser channels. They found that MAL diffused 1.5 mm from each laser channel. As more is learned about how far each agent studied diffuses, it will allow for optimal channel density. Of course every drug, cell, and cosmeceuticals diffusion will be based on its inherent properties. Physiochemical properties including size of molecule, diffusion coefficient, skin disease, and other factors affect the ability of different compounds to transverse tissue.

As much as been learned to date about laser dosimetry for LAD of drugs the interaction of the laser parameters will need to be studied and customized for each individual drug or device.

Laser-Assisted Delivery Facial Scar Technique

The majority of treatments are performed in office using topical anesthetic preparations under occlusion for 1 hour or more before treatment. Selected pulse energies are proportional to the scar thickness. Higher pulse energy settings recommend lower treatment densities of 5% to 10%. The treatment area includes the entire scar sheet and a 1- to 2-mm rim of normal skin. Within 2 minutes of stopping the laser, the drug or device is applied topically or injected in the needed area. Then, immediately after ablative fractional treatments and laser-assisted drug delivery is completed, petrolatum or a petrolatum-based ointment is applied and continued several times daily until the site is fully epithelialized, usually within 3 or 4 days. Patients may resume showering the following day and begin gentle daily cleansing with mild soap of the area at least twice a day. Patients are allowed to resume essentially normal activity after treatment. Oral antibiotics and antivirals are commonly used for prophylaxis starting 1 day before treatment and continuing for up to 1 week. Antifungal agents may be entertained on a case-by-case basis or if the patient develops localized pain or pruritus after laser treatment. When treating facial areas, viral prophylaxis should be considered. Photoprotection should be advocated, including avoidance in the early posttreatment period and application of bland sun blocks (zinc or titanium dioxide) once epithelial integrity is restored and for 12 weeks after laser therapy.

As discussed, scar therapy takes a multidisciplinary, multimodal approach for optimal success. Before, during, and after LAD therapy, other specialists including reconstructive surgeons, physical therapists, occupational therapists, and psychiatrists also treat the patient. In cases of scar contracture, participation in physical and occupational therapy is highly recommended to take full advantage of the laser effects. Compression therapy while healing from LAD with either silicone gel sheets, tight athletic wear, and/or medical compression garments.

Agents for Laser-Assisted Delivery Systems for Treatment of Facial Scars

In scars, laser ablated zones may be used immediately to deliver drugs and other substances to synergistically create an enhanced therapeutic response. Ablative channels are generally 100 to 4000 microns in depth for targeted cutaneous drug delivery. By combining laser therapy with drugs, molecules, or devices simultaneously we may achieve a more optimal clinical result in scars.

LASER-ASSISTED DELIVERY TREATMENT OF EXISTING FACIAL SCARS

Laser alone can be effective treatment of facial scars. When a drug, molecule, or device that has appropriate properties is added to the ablative channels, there is a synergistic improvement in the scar that cannot be obtained from either the laser or the drug alone. This section reviews various approaches to treating existing facial scars with LAD.

Hypertrophic Facial Scars: Laser-Assisted Delivery of Triamcinolone Acetonide and 5-Fluorouracil

Ablative fractional laser-assisted delivery has been used to treat hypertrophic scars (**Figs. 2–4**). Triamcinolone acetonide immediately after fractional laser takes advantage of the ablative fractional laser's ability to penetrate deep into the hypertrophic scars and synergistically decrease collagen. In a human study performed using laser assisted drug delivery of triamcinolone acetonide to improve scars, Waibel and colleagues[27] evaluated in a prospective, single-arm, pilot study including 15 consecutive subjects with hypertrophic scars from burns, trauma, and surgery. Subjects underwent 3 to 5 treatment sessions at 2- to 3-month intervals consisting of postoperative topical application of triamcinolone acetonide solution at a concentration of 10 mg/mL. The objective of this study was to evaluate the efficacy and safety of a new combination therapy that incorporates ablative fractional CO_2 laser in the same treatment session as topical triamcinolone acetonide to synergistically improve complicated scars. Combination same session laser therapy resulted in average overall improvement of 2.73/3.0. However, corticosteroids have the potential to cause several adverse events, including dermal atrophy, fat atrophy, hyperpigmentation, telangiectasia, and hypopigmentation. In another study, Issa and colleagues[28] used ultrasound technology in addition to fractional ablative radiofrequency therapy to assist in the delivery of triamcinolone in hypertrophic scars of 4 patients. The objective was to evaluate clinical response and side effect of LAD technology in hypertrophic scars in the body and face using ablative fractional radiofrequency associated with low-frequency acoustic pressure ultrasound therapy. This research concluded ablative fractional radiofrequency associated with acoustic pressure ultrasound therapy could improve the efficacy of steroids in hypertrophic scar treatment, minimizing the risks of localized atrophy and irregular appearance of the treated lesion.

Intralesional 5-FU is a safe and effective intralesional treatment of scars.[28] Although there are systemic toxicity concerns, LAD of 5-FU may have benefits over LAD of corticosteroid. Waibel and colleagues[28] also studied LADS of 5-FU

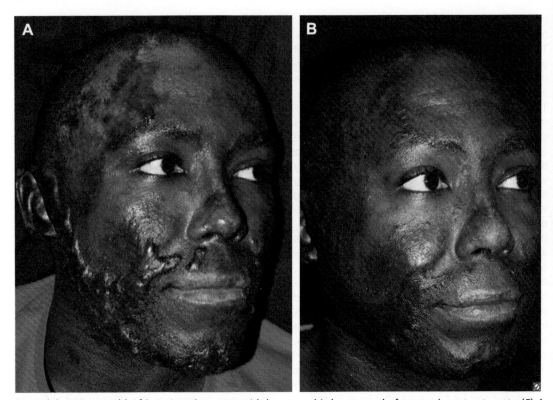

Fig. 2. (*A*) A 41-year-old African American man with hypertrophic burn scars before any laser treatments. (*B*) A 41-year-old African American man with hypertrophic burn scars after fractional ablative laser, along with laser-assisted delivery of triamcinolone acetonide injections.

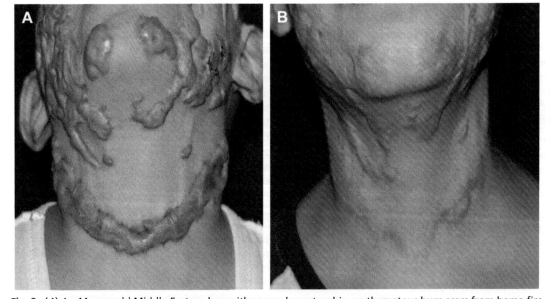

Fig. 3. (*A*) An 11-year-old Middle Eastern boy with severe hypertrophic, erythematous burn scars from home fire before any treatment. (*B*) An 11-year-old Middle Eastern boy with severe hypertrophic, erythematous home fire burn scars after 3 treatments with ablative fractional laser, nonablative fractional lasers, along with laser-assisted delivery of triamcinolone acetonide.

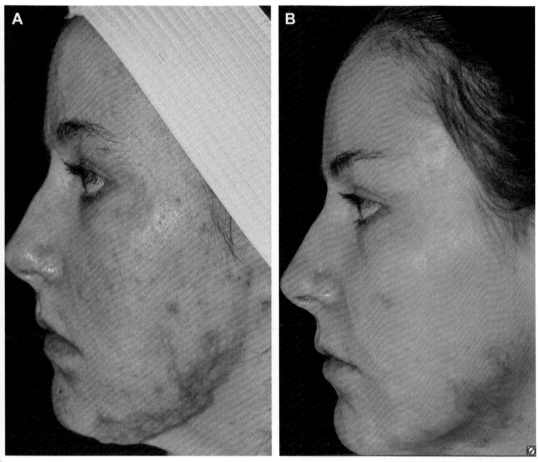

Fig. 4. (*A*) A 22-year-old Caucasian woman with erythematous, hypetrophic burn scars from a bonfire before any treatment. (*B*) A 22-year-old Caucasian woman with erythematous, hypertrophic bonfire burn scars after fractional ablative lasers, nonablative fractional ablative lasers, along with laser-assisted delivery of 5-fluoracil.

versus triamcinolone acetonide for hypertrophic scar treatment. LAD with fractional ablative laser was studied to deliver 5-FU versus triamcinolone acetonide solution to synergistically create an enhanced therapeutic response when treating human hypertrophic scars. The study evaluated using LAD in a head-to-head trial on 2 separate but similar scars with triamcinolone acetonide solution or 5-FU solution on the same patient. Results indicate equal efficacy of the 2 agents for decreasing scar height and length; however, triamcinolone acetonide had more adverse events including increased width and increased telangiectasia.

Atrophic Facial Scars and Laser-Assisted Delivery of Poly-L-Lactic Acid

Atrophic scars represent a significant loss of collagen upon healing. Fractional lasers are known to be effective in the treatment of atrophic scars.[29] Poly-L-lactic acid (PLLA) is a tissue stimulator that

is typically injected into the subcutaneous or supraperiosteal plane for the purpose of facial volume correction. LAD of PLLA combined with the properties of fractional ablative resurfacing stimulates fibroblast proliferation and neocollagenesis (**Fig. 5**). This study was a prospective, uncontrolled of the treatment of 19 patients with atrophic scars with ablative fractional CO_2 laser and topically applied 0.5 mL PLLA. The laser settings depth from 375 to 500 microns and a density of 10%. The PLLA was reconstituted at least 24 hours in advance and diluted with 6 mL of sterile saline and 2 mL of 1% lidocaine HCL with epinephrine at a concentration of 1:100,000 to evaluate the ablative fractional laser on the patient's skin and migration of the PLLA into the columns fresh human cadaver cheek. Four blinded dermatologist first identified before and after photographs. The average overall improvement score was 2.18 on a scale of 0 to 3. Of the 20 photographs, 65% had an improvement score of 2.0 or greater. The

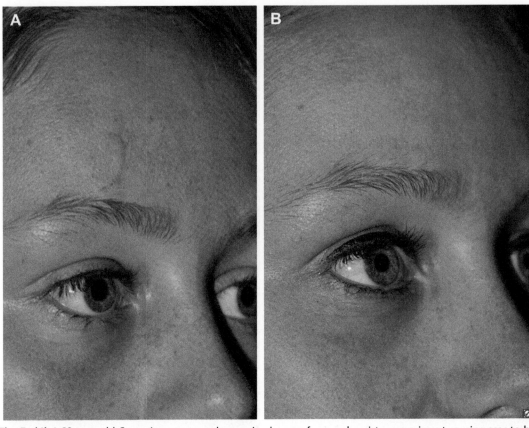

Fig. 5. (*A*) A 22-year-old Caucasian woman who received a scar from a chemistry experiment causing scar to be atrophic. (*B*) A 22-year-old Caucasian woman after 1 treatment of fractional ablative laser along with laser-assisted delivery of poly-L-lactic acid.

cadaver pathology showed evidence using polarized light to demonstrate PLLA in the channels created by the laser.

Hypopigmented Facial Scars: Bimatoprost

Hypopigmentation is a common problem in scar patients after surgical, acne, burn, and trauma scars. Improving hypopigmentation has been a medical challenge owing to the limited treatment options. Hypopigmentation can be a significant issue in patients with skin of color. In prior studies, it has been shown that many hypopigmented skin conditions have inactive melanocytes that may be stimulated to produce pigment. Possible ways to create pigment in hypopigmented skin includes the use of laser only, LAD of bimatoprost, and melanocyte transplantation using a novel epidermal harvesting system.

Recently, fractional laser has been demonstrated to produce improvement in hypopigmentation of acne and surgical scars. The mechanism of action is hypothesized to be repopulation of melanocytes in hypopigmented areas from surrounding hair follicles and basal melanocytes.

Bimatoprost is a drug brought to market to treat glaucoma and was noted to have a side effect that could cause periocular hyperpigmentation owing to increased melanogenesis. There seems to be a dose-dependent relationship and mechanism for increased melanogenesis and increased transfer of melanosomes with the absence of melanocyte atypia (**Fig. 6**).

In the LAD of the bimatoprost arm, immediately after fractional ablative laser therapy topical bimatoprost 0.03% is placed over hypopigmented scars. Patients are instructed to apply the product twice a day until they use all of it. In this case, because melanocytes are superficial, superficial laser ablative settings are needed.[30,31]

Laser-assisted delivery synergistically acute injury or wound: Improve wound healing or prevent scarring

Wound healing: laser-assisted delivery vitamins C and E and ferulic acid In a split face comparison, the effects of vitamin CE ferulic acid formula (Skinceuticals, New York, NY) immediately after fractional ablative laser pretreatment to

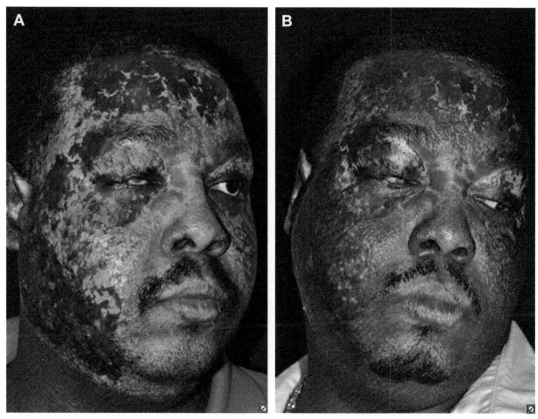

Fig. 6. (*A*) A 41-year-old African American man with hypopigmented scars from a chemical burn before any treatment. (*B*) A 41-year-old African American man after 5 fractional ablative laser treatments along with laser-assisted delivery with bimatoprost topical application on chemical burn scars.

decrease postoperative recovery and increase neo-collagenosis in fractional ablative laser resurfacing for photodamage was performed. Secondary objectives were to evaluate synergistic response of laser and topical application on the upregulation and formation of collagen through histologic evaluation of messenger RNA and collagens I and III. Previous studies have shown that application of vitamins C and E, and ferulic acid improves wound healing and promotes the induction of collagen.[19] The objective of this study was to prospectively evaluate the efficacy of vitamins C and E, and ferulic acid, decreasing postoperative downtime. Secondary objectives were to evaluate synergistic response of laser and topical application on the up regulation and formation of collagen through histologic evaluation of messenger RNA and collagens I and III. Results from this study showed trends of decreasing downtime 24 to 48 hours with patients able to return to work and social life more quickly.

Atrophic and hypopigmented facial wounds: Laser-assisted delivery epidermal skin transplantation A novel device currently used to perform epidermal

grafting procedures is a donor site sparing harvesting system, which enables the transfer of autologous epidermis that includes live melanocytes. This epidermal harvesting system technology creates microsuction blisters known as microdomes by using a combination of vacuum and warmth. This tool allows for epidermal skin grafting in the outpatient setting without donor site morbidities like scarring (**Fig. 7**).

The novel epidermal harvesting technology procedure begins with donor site preparation (removal of hair then wiped with alcohol). The donor site is typically the inner thigh, an area with limited sun exposure and a melanocyte-rich area of the body. The harvester is placed on the donor site then vacuum and warmth are applied via the CelluTome control unit. In approximately 30 minutes, the autologous epidermal microblisters are formed. Recipient site preparation with fractional ablative CO_2 laser at superficial depth can occur during microdome formation for procedural efficiency. The epidermal graft acquisition occurs once the transfer dressing is positioned onto the microdomes. Once harvested, a

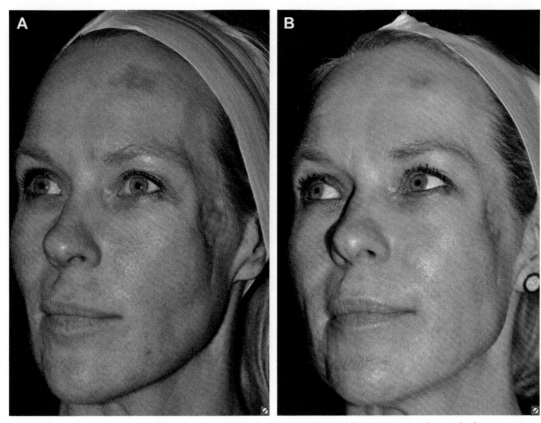

Fig. 7. (*A*) A 48-year-old Caucasian woman with severely atrophic and hypopigmented scars before any treatment. (*B*) A 48-year-old Caucasian woman with severely atrophic, and hypopigmented scars after 1 fractional ablative treatments along with an epidermal harvesting system.

ready-to-apply Tegaderm array of autologous epidermal micrografts is transferred to the prepared recipient hypopigmented sites. Donor sites are covered for 24 hours after procedure with Tegaderm. The recipient site will be covered with hypofix for 3 to 5 days after procedure.

What is the best technique to enhance laser-assisted delivery?

Topical application/topical application with occlusion/acoustic device/meretes article/gel matrix model Given the established benefit with laser ablation, there is now growing belief that using energy driven methods may enhance drug delivery in a synergistic manner. Processes such as iontophoresis, electroporation, sonophoresis, and the use of photomechanical waves all provide various ways to aid in penetration. Sonophoresis, the use of ultrasound technology to enhance the transport of a substance through a liquid medium, is particularly interesting given the emerging role for ultrasound technology in dermatology. Energy is delivered to the ultrasonic horn by an ultrasonic control system at a frequency of approximately

30 kHz. The force of cavitation causes the formation of holes in the corneocytes, enlarging of intercellular spaces, and perturbation of stratum corneum lipids. The increase in temperature increases the fluidity of the stratum corneum lipids as well directly increasing the diffusivity of molecules through the skin barrier.[4,20]

A transdermal sonophoresis delivery system has been developed to enhance the delivery of topical cosmeceuticals. This device has frequency up to 100 Hz and peak power of 40 W. The hypothesis is that this device emits acoustic waves and air pressure, which pushes active components deeper into the skin and helps to promote topical absorption when paired with LAD to enhance penetration. Five patients were treated and biopsied with 4 treatment sites—1 area treated with topically applied ALA, 1 area with fractional ablative laser and ALA topically applied, 1 area with fractional ablative laser and transdermal delivery system, and 1 area of ALA topically applied with transdermal delivery system. Comparison of the difference of magnitude of diffusion both lateral spread of ALA and depth diffusion of ALA will be measured by fluorescence microscopy. With laser plus ALA plus an acoustic device, the protoporphyrin IX lateral fluorescence was 0.024 mm on average versus fractional laser and ALA only was 0.0084. The diffusion with the acoustic air device was an order of magnitude greater. In our prospective study, we found that our combined approach of fractional CO_2 laser and the acoustic air device gave us the best results of the increased depth of penetration of the ALA.

Another study by Erlendsson and colleagues[32] sought to investigate a standardized method to actively fill laser-generated channels by altering pressure, vacuum, and pressure (PVP), studying effect on (i) relative filling of individual laser channels, (ii) cutaneous deposition and delivery kinetics, and (iii) biodistribution and diffusion pattern, estimated by mathematical simulation.

The results revealed that active filling with application of PVP increased the number of filled laser channels. At a depth of 1000 μm, filling increased from 44% (AFXL) to 94% with 1 PVP cycle (AFXL + PVP; P <.01). Active filling greatly enhanced intracutaneous deposition of PEG400, resulting in a rapid delivery 6-folding uptake at 10 minutes (AFXL 54 μg/mL vs AFXL + PVP 303 μg/mL; P <.01). This study concluded that active filling with PVP filling of laser channels induces a deeper, greater, more rapid delivery than ablative fractional laser alone.

Limitations of laser-assisted delivery

Overall, fractional ablative lasers have a favorable adverse event rate.[33] Of course there are also concomitant risks of the drug, cosmeceutical, or other substance applied to the skin that also must be taken into account. Theoretically, any drug may be used in LAD; however, the US Food and Drug Administration–approved uses of the drug, physiochemical properties of drug, target tissue, lost drug, and cost must be considered. In addition, it must be noted that not all drugs were meant or studied to be put down into the dermis. Drugs and cosmeceuticals studied only for epidermal purposes may have untoward effects if placed in the dermis and systemic circulation. As more studies are reported, we will find conditions and compounds that will benefit the most from LAD. Scars seem to be 1 condition that have responded favorably to LAD. Another potential drawback of LAD using fractional ablative CO_2 or Er:YAG system is that the cost of these devices usually thousands of dollars. Another laser drawback is owing to the ablative wounds there is a minimal 1 to 2 day healing time and mild discomfort with the procedure.

Safety concerns

Because the dermal channels have direct access to the vascular system, there are concerns of potential systemic toxicity. In addition, lasers also create a direct entry for bacteria and other pathogens directly to the blood supply. Oni and colleagues[19] also studied that laser pretreatment significantly increased absorption of topical lidocaine to levels detectable in the blood.

Cushing's syndrome has been reported in post burn children after intralesional triamcinolone injection.[34] Cushing's syndrome after intralesional administration of triamcinolone acetate has been reported twice, both in adult patients. This paper reports on 2 pediatric cases of Cushing's syndrome after treatment of hypertrophic burn scars with intralesional triamcinolone acetonide. Intralesional triamcinolone acetate therapy was initiated 3 months after a burn injury and in neither child was the maximum recommended dose exceeded. In both children, Cushing's manifestations developed 1 to 2 weeks after injection and resolved in 6 to 8 weeks with no treatment or permanent sequelae. It seems that these 2 pediatric patients may have had a form of hypersensitivity to triamcinolone acetonide, because the Cushing's syndrome was not the result of an overdose. Systemic effects include liver toxicity and Cushing's syndrome.

SUMMARY

Ablative fractional lasers offer a unique therapeutic modality to destroy stratum corneum, epidermal, and dermal layers of the skin in a predictable and controlled manner for the delivery of topically applied molecules. There remain many questions, including ideal fluences, densities, and drug concentrations. Each indication used for LAD will need extensive research for optimization. Many drugs are not intended for use in the dermis and so it yet to be determined which drugs are appropriate for LAD. It seems this emerging technology has the ability to be a new delivery system for both localized and systemic delivery of drugs, cells, and other bioactive agents. As research continues, we will learn the most efficient approach to deliver substances whether it is a topical approach, occlusion, PVP, acoustic wave, or gel matrix. With responsible development, ablative fractional laser-assisted drug delivery may become a new important part of facial scar therapy.

REFERENCES

1. Anderson RR, Donelan MB, Hivnor C, et al. Laser treatment of traumatic scars with an emphasis on

ablative fractional laser resurfacing consensus report. JAMA Dermatol 2014;150(2):187–93.

2. Waibel J, Wulkan A, Lupo M, et al. Treatment of burn scars with the 1550 nm nonablative fractional erbium laser. Lasers Surg Med 2012;44:44.

3. Sklar L, Burnett C, Waibel J, et al. Laser assisted drug delivery: a review of an evolving technology. Lasers Surg Med 2014;9999:1–14.

4. Haedersdal M, Sakamoto FH, Farinelli WA, et al. Fractional CO_2 laser-assisted drug delivery. Lasers Surg Med 2010;42:113–22.

5. Bloom B, Brauer J, Geronemus R. Ablative fractional resurfacing in topical drug delivery: an update and outlook. Dermatol Surg 2013;39:839–48.

6. Yun PL, Tchihara R, Anderson RR. Efficacy of erbium:yttrium-aluminum-garnet laser-assisted delivery of topical anesthetic. J Am Acad Dermatol 2002;47(4):542–7.

7. Haak CS, Farinelli WA, Tam J, et al. Fractional laser-assisted delivery of methyl aminolevulinate: impact of laser channel depth and incubation time. Lasers Surg Med 2012;44(10):787–95.

8. Asilian A, Darougheh A, Shariati F. New combination of triamcinolone, 5-fluorouracil, and pulsed-dye laser for treatment of keloid and hypertrophic scars. Dermatol Surg 2006;32(7):907–15.

9. Hsiao CY, Huang CH, Hu S, et al. Fractional carbon dioxide laser treatment to enhance skin permeation of ascorbic acid 2-glucoside with minimal skin disruption. Dermatol Surg 2012;38(8):1284–93.

10. Marra DE, Yip D, Fincher EF, et al. Systemic toxicity from topically applied lidocaine in conjunction with fractional photothermolysis. Arch Dermatol 2006;142(8):1024–6.

11. Lee WR, Shen SC, Al-Suwayeh SA, et al. Laser-assisted topical drug delivery by using a low-fluence fractional laser: imiquimod and macromolecules. J Control Release 2011;153(3):240–8.

12. Lee WR, Pan TL, Wang PW, et al. Erbium:YAG laser enhances transdermal peptide delivery and skin vaccination. J Control Release 2008;128(3):200–8.

13. Gomez C, Costela A, Garcia-Moreno I, et al. Laser treatments on skin enhancing and controlling transdermal delivery of 5-fluorouracil. Lasers Surg Med 2008;40(1):6–12.

14. Lee WR, Shen SC, Fang CL, et al. Topical delivery of methotrexate via skin pretreated with physical enhancement techniques: low-fluence erbium:YAG laser and electroporation. Lasers Surg Med 2008;40(7):468–76.

15. Forster B, Klein A, Szeimies RM, et al. Penetration enhancement of two topical 5-aminolaevulinic acid formulations for photodynamic therapy by erbium:YAG laser ablation of the stratum corneum: continuous versus fractional ablation. Exp Dermatol 2010;19(9):806–12.

16. Erlendsson AM, Taudorf EH, Eriksson AH, et al. Ablative fractional laser alters biodistribution of ingenol mebutate in the skin. Arch Dermatol Res 2015;307(6):515–22.

17. Bachhav YG, Heinrich A, Kaila YN. Using laser microporation to improve transdermal delivery of diclofenac: increasing bioavailability and the range of therapeutic applications. Eur J Pharm Biopharm 2011;78(3):408–14.

18. Oni G, Brown SA, Kenkel JM. Can fractional lasers enhance transdermal absorption of topical lidocaine in an in vivo animal model? Lasers Surg Med 2012;44(2):168–74.

19. Waibel J, Mi QS, Ozog D, et al. Laser assisted delivery of vitamin C, vitamin E, and Ferulic acid formula serum decreases fractional laser post-operative recovery by increased beta fibroblast growth factor expression. Lasers Surg Med 2016;48(3):238–44.

20. Waibel JS, Badiavas E. A pilot study of laser assisted drug delivery of allogenic mesenchymal cutaneous stem cells resulting in functional chimeric mouse model. ASLMS; 2012.

21. Kim H, Gallo J. Evaluation of the effect of platelet-rich plasma on recovery after ablative fractional photothermolysis. JAMA Facial Plast Surg 2015;17(2):97–102.

22. Haedersdal M, Erlendsson A, Paasch U, et al. Traditional medicine in the field of ablative fractional laser (AFXL) – assisted drug delivery: a critical review from basics to current clinical status. J Am Acad Dermatol 2016;74(5):981–1004.

23. Bachhav YG, Summer S, Heinrich A, et al. Effect of controlled laser microporation on drug transport kinetics into and across the skin. J Control Release 2010;146:31–6.

24. Sakamoto F, Wanner M, Farinelli W, et al. Aminolevulinic acid photodynamic therapy (ALA-PDT) delivered after ablative fractional resurfacing in an animal model. Lasers Surg Med 2009;41 [abstract: 79].

25. Haak C, Bhayana B, Farinelli W, et al. Fractional CO2 laser assisted drug delivery is affected by laser density and molecular weight. Lasers Surg Med 2012;44:36–7.

26. Haedersdal M, Katsnelson J, Sakamoto FH, et al. Enhanced uptake and photoactivation of topical methyl aminolevulinate after fractional CO_2 laser pretreatment. Lasers Surg Med 2011;43:804–13.

27. Waibel JS, Wulkan AJ, Shumaker PR. Treatment of hypertrophic scars using laser and laser assisted corticosteroid delivery. Lasers Surg Med 2013;45:135–40.

28. Issa MC, Kassuga LE, Chevrand NS, et al. Topical delivery of triamcinolone via skin pretreated with ablative radiofrequency: a new method in hypertrophic scar treatment. Int J Dermatol 2013;52(3):367–70.

29. Rkein A, Ozog D, Waibel JS. Treatment of atrophic scars with fractionated CO2 laser facilitating delivery of topically applied poly-L-Lactic acid. Dermatol Surg 2014;0:1–8.

30. Massaki A, Fabi S, Fitzpatrick R. Repigmentation of hypopigmented scars using an erbium-Doped 1,550 nm fractionated laser and topical bimatoprost. Dermatol Surg 2012;38:995–1001.

31. Erlendsson AM, Anderson RR, Manstein D, et al. Developing technology: ablative fractional lasers enhance topical drug delivery. Dermatol Surg 2014;40(Suppl 12):S142–6.

32. Erlendsson AM, Doukas AG, Farinelli WA, et al. Fractional laser-assisted drug delivery: active filling of laser channels with pressure and vacuum alteration. Lasers Surg Med 2016;48(2):116–24.

33. Metelitsa AI, Alster TS. Fractionated laser skin resurfacing treatment complications: a review. Dermatol Surg 2010;36:299–306.

34. Ritota PC, Lo AK. Cushing's syndrome in postburn children following intralesional triamcinolone injection. Ann Plast Surg 1996;36(5):508–11.

Skin Color and Pigmentation in Ethnic Skin

Marty O. Visscher, PhD

KEYWORDS

- Skin type • Skin color • Pigmentation • Ethnicity • Melanocyte • Ultraviolet radiation
- Individual typology angle • Hyperpigmentation

KEY POINTS

- Skin color classification is a cornerstone of clinical practice. Quantitation of pigmentation in the context of response to stress is essential for determining cutaneous treatments.
- The quantity and distribution of melanin-producing melanocytes varies with inherent skin color. Both individually distributed and clustered melanosomes are significantly larger in African versus white skin, and of intermediate size in Asians.
- The greatest increase in melanosome protein levels after ultraviolet exposure occurred in black people. The melanin distribution varied with skin color, moving from the lower to middle layers and to a greater extent in black skin.
- Genetic studies across pigmentation types have identified at least 120 genes associated with skin pigmentation and the melanocortin 1 receptor gene seems to predominate.
- The relationship between ancestry/ethnicity and skin pigmentation shows a significant but modest correlation and high variability.

INTRODUCTION

Human skin color uniformity and distribution communicate physiologic health status.[1] Facial images with uniform skin coloration are judged as younger versus images with highly variable color.[2] For example, individuals were asked to adjust the red color component of facial images until it represented a healthy appearance. All observers increased red color but dark-skinned observers increased the redness of dark skin images more than for lighter skin images.[3] Japanese women with darker and more yellow skin color were classified as older.[4] This article discusses skin color, pigmentation, and ethnicity as they relate to clinical practice. Color perception, skin typing/classification, and quantitation are reviewed in relation to ethnicity, environmental stresses/irritants, and potential treatment effects.

COLOR PERCEPTION

Humans detect color when retinal cone cells receive and mediate light via peak absorption at 564 to 580 nm (red), 534 to 545 nm (green), and 420 to 440 nm (blue) wavelengths of the color spectrum.[5,6] Visible light interacts with skin components; namely, melanins (yellow to black), oxygenated hemoglobin (red), deoxyhemoglobin (blue-purple), bilirubin (yellow), and carotene (yellow).[7] Approximately 5% is reflected back and the remainder is transmitted, absorbed, or scattered.[2] The stratum corneum transmits light. The epidermis and dermis absorb light because of melanin and hemoglobin. Melanin is synthesized by the melanocytes and transferred to keratinocytes throughout the epidermis.[8] Oxygenated blood (dermal capillaries, vascular plexus) and deoxygenated blood (dermal venules) contribute

Funding Source: None.
Conflict of Interest: None.
Skin Sciences Program, Cincinnati, OH, USA
E-mail address: Marty.visscher@gmail.com

Facial Plast Surg Clin N Am 25 (2017) 119–125
http://dx.doi.org/10.1016/j.fsc.2016.08.011

facialplastic.theclinics.com

to skin color.[9] Epidermal carotene and bilirubin contribute to yellow coloration. Bilirubin is deposited in phospholipid membranes and leaked into extravascular regions.[10] Light is scattered within the epidermis, dermis, and subcutaneous fat.[11]

Two kinds of skin pigmentation are considered here. Constitutive pigmentation is the inherent type; that is, the color of sun-protected areas such as the upper inner arm (**Table 1**). Facultative pigmentation is produced as a result of ultraviolet (UV) exposure, either chronically or in response to a specific dose of radiation. Facultative pigmentation varies for an individual, reflecting changes in UV intensity with changes in season. Minimal erythema dose (MED) is the minimum amount of ultraviolet radiation required to produce minimum erythema (see **Table 1**).

Skin pigmentation protects living cells from the injurious effects of environmental UV radiation and repairs the DNA damage that occurs.[12] Epidermal melanin diminishes UV penetration and removes reactive oxygen species generated during UV exposure.[13] UV radiation can suppress the immune system's ability to prevent actions of tumor antigens both systemically and locally, as shown by changes in and reduction of the levels of Langerhans cells.[14,15] Constitutive pigmentation varies in the effectiveness of the protection it affords living cells.

SKIN COLOR CLASSIFICATION

Skin color classification is a cornerstone of clinical practice and is used to decide on the treatment of cutaneous conditions. The Fitzpatrick skin type system originated in 1975 from a need to better predict patient response to the UVA radiation used in psoriasis treatment.[16] Patients of similar visual skin color reacted differently to the same UVA dose, with some developing severe burns. The classification was broadened to include response to environmental stress, namely UV radiation. Therefore, the UV response serves as a surrogate for predicting the reactivity to other stresses, such as laser energy. Inherent skin coloration (constitutive pigmentation) and reaction to UV radiation (facultative pigmentation) gave rise to 6 types. Fitzpatrick phototype I always burns, never tans; phototype II usually burns, sometimes tans; phototype III may burn, usually tans; phototype IV rarely burns, always tans; phototype V has moderate constitutional pigmentation; and phototype VI has marked constitutional pigmentation.[17] Total UV exposure is associated with the incidence of squamous cell carcinoma, which is higher in light skin and high reactivity to UV radiation.[18] The lightest skin types experience the highest incidence of melanoma.[19]

Limitations of the Fitzpatrick system have been noted, because of difficulties with self-reports of the effects of UV exposure.[20] The relationship between self-assessed Fitzpatrick type and skin color at the wrist (sun protected) was determined among 3386 ethnically diverse subjects. The darkest Fitzpatrick types (V and VI) were self-assigned in 17.7% of participants with the lightest skin.[21] Statistical modeling showed the selected Fitzpatrick type to be 1 classification off, on average. To address these limitations, a color-based method for skin type self-assessment was developed from evaluations of 120 white, Hispanic, and African people. They selected their skin coloration from a color figure (available at www.jaad.org) and questions about effects of UV exposure. Melanin index was measured spectroscopically.[22] Efforts to develop more objective, quantitative skin color measurements to assist clinicians in predicting response to skin treatments are ongoing.

Table 1
Melanin content for unexposed skin by classification

Classification	Melanin Content (μg/mg)
Ethnic Group	
Asian	3.9
Black/African American	15
Hispanic/Latin American	8
Native Hawaiian/other Pacific Islander	11
White	4.5
Fitzpatrick Skin Phototype	
1 and 2	4
2.5	5
3 and 3.5	5.7
4	11.5
4.6–6	13
MED Range (J/m^2)	
$\leq$225	3.5
226–300	4
301–400	7.3
401–600	9.5
601–800	12.3
$\geq$801	14.3

Abbreviation: MED, minimal erythema dose.
From Tadokoro T, Kobayashi N, Zmudzka BZ, et al. UV-induced DNA damage and melanin content in human skin differing in racial/ethnic origin. FASEB J 2003;17:1177–9; with permission.

Quantitation of Skin Color

Expert visual assessment of skin color is routine in clinical practice but is limited by high variation and low reliability.[23,24] Digital imaging (standardized lighting, focal length, positioning, color correction) and spectroscopic methods have been used to improve objectivity and to quantify features (eg, dyspigmentation, erythema).[11,25,26] Digital photographs (collected as RGB, ie, red, green, blue colors), are typically converted to L*a*b* color (L*, lightness-darkness; a*, red-green; and b*, yellow-blue) because it better replicates human color perception.[6,27,28]

The impact of melanin on lightness (L*), red-green (a*), and blue-yellow (b*) as a function of ethnicity (European, Chinese, Mexican, Indian, African) was investigated in the experiments by Alaluf and colleagues.[29] For sun-protected skin sites, lightness was highest for Europeans and lowest for Africans. Indian skin was significantly darker than European, Chinese, and Mexican skin. Red color (a*) was significantly higher for Indian and African versus the other groups. Yellow color (b*) was significantly higher for Indian and African versus all others and for Chinese and Mexican versus European. L* was significantly and inversely correlated with levels of eumelanin and total melanin overall and for all ethnic groups (correlation coefficients, −0.77 to 0.89). Although significant, L* was inversely correlated with pheomelanin amounts with lower correlations (−0.23; range, −0.53 to 0.83).

To quantify pigmentation, the individual typology angle (ITA) was determined from L* and b* values using this equation:

$$ITA = [arctan(L*-50)/b*)]*180/\pi, \text{ where } \pi = 3.14.$$

The values constitute 6 groups of skin pigmentation: ITA greater than 55° (very light), 41° to 55° (light), 28° to 41° (intermediate), 10° to 28° (tan), −30° to 10° (brown), and less than−30° (dark).[7] The ITA values and categories, shown in **Fig. 1**, were reported for 3500 subjects from white, African, Asian, Hispanic, and Brazilian ethnic groups.[30] ITA values correlated with skin pigmentation.[31] Skin erythema, with confounders from perfusion, is typically quantified by a* color value. **Fig. 2** shows the ITA values (see **Fig. 2A**) for each ethnicity, along with eumelanin and pheomelanin levels (see **Fig. 2B**) from Alaluf and colleagues[29] (described earlier). The associations among skin classifications are shown in **Fig. 3** along with corresponding melanin index ranges (spectroscopic assessment),[32] minimum erythema dose ranges,[33] and colors typified by each classification.[34]

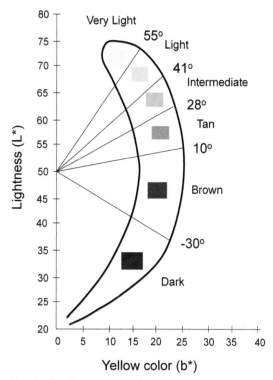

Fig. 1. The 6 categories of skin coloration from very light to dark and the accompanying ITA values. Skin lightness is plotted versus yellow color (b*). The lines show the angles for each classification. Higher ITA values indicate lighter skin. Individual values are typically plotted for population studies, as reported for 3500 subjects encompassing white, African, Asian, Hispanic, and Brazilian ethnic groups. (*Adapted from* Del Bino S, Sok J, Bessac E, et al. Relationship between skin response to ultraviolet exposure and skin color type. Pigment Cell Res 2006;19:606–14; with permission; and *Data from* Del Bino S, Bernerd F. Variations in skin colour and the biological consequences of ultraviolet radiation exposure. Br J Dermatol 2013;169(Suppl 3):33–40.)

CAUSES OF SKIN COLOR VARIATION
Physiology

Variation in constitutive pigmentation is caused by differences in the amount and type of melanin in the basal epidermis.[35] Melanin is synthesized in organelles, melanosomes, located in melanocytes residing in the basal epidermis and transferred to keratinocytes throughout the epidermis.[8] Melanosomes contain enzymes (eg, dopachrome tautomerase) and structural proteins that synthesize melanin.[36] Although their density does not vary with inherent skin color, the quantity and distribution of melanocytes differ.[37]

Two melanin types, eumelanin (brown-black) and pheomelanin (yellow-red), contribute to color.[38] Eumelanin protects from UV damage.[39] On UV exposure, pheomelanin produces more free

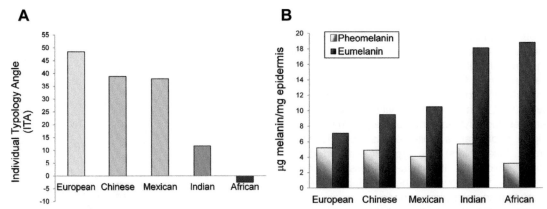

Fig. 2. ITA values (*A*) and melanin levels (*B*) for European, Chinese, Mexican, Indian, and African people. Lightness (sun protected) was highest for Europeans and lowest for Africans. Indian skin was significantly darker than European, Chinese, and Mexican skin. L^* was significantly and inversely correlated with levels of eumelanin and total melanin overall and for all groups (correlation coefficients, -0.77 to 0.89 for both total melanin and eumelanin). Although significant, L^* was inversely correlated with pheomelanin levels with lower correlations (-0.23 overall ranging from -0.53 to 0.83). (*Data from* Alaluf S, Atkins D, Barrett K, et al. The impact of epidermal melanin on objective measurements of human skin colour. Pigment Cell Res 2002;15:119–26.)

radicals ($^1O_2$) over a longer time than eumelanin, thereby producing more damage.[40] Pheomelanin levels are higher in phenotypes with fair skin and red hair.[18] Melanin characteristics and skin lightness were examined among European, Chinese, Mexican, Indian (continental India), and African subjects.[41] European skin was the lightest and not statistically different from Chinese and Mexican. Indian and Africans had significantly darker skin. For all groups, lightness was higher for sun-protected versus sun-exposed skin. Melanin levels (constitutive, sun protected) were higher in Indian and Black skin versus European, Chinese and Mexican. Pheomelanin level decreased as the skin darkened, except for Indian subjects, in whom pheomelanin levels were higher than in Mexican and Chinese subjects (see **Fig. 2**B). Eumelanin level increased with darkening; that is, Indian and African subjects had more than Mexican, Chinese, and European subjects (see **Fig. 2**B). Pheomelanin levels were higher in sun-protected areas versus sun-exposed sites. The concentration of spheroidal melanosomes was higher in sun-protected sites across groups. Melanosome size was smaller in sun-protected versus sun-exposed samples. Melanosome size increased as the skin darkened; that is, smaller in European and larger in African skin.

Melanosome distribution and size within the keratinocytes of tissues from African, Asian, and white ethnicities were examined by quantitative microscopy. Melanosomes were distributed individually throughout the cells, usually over the nuclei, in African skin.[42] They were in membrane-bound clusters in white skin and showed an intermediate distribution in Asian skin. Melanosome

sizes varied with distribution pattern for Asians; individual melanosomes were larger than clustered melanosomes. Both individually distributed and clustered melanosomes were significantly larger in African versus white skin and of intermediate sizes in Asian skin. Sizes for Asian versus white melanosomes were statistically different, whereas Asian versus African sizes were not.

Mechanism of Constitutive Pigmentation Control

The potential mechanisms involved in determining constitutive pigmentation were investigated by generating cell cultures of melanocytes, keratinocytes, and fibroblasts from light-skinned and dark-skinned foreskins and grafting them onto immunocompromised mice using implantation

Fitzpatrick Type	UVB MED mJ/cm^2	Melanin Index Range	ITA Range
I	20–30	9000–10550	>55
II	25–35	8600–9400	42–55
III	30–50	8000–8830	35–41
IV	45–60	6200–7050	29–34
V	60–100	4800–5600	21–28
VI	100–200	3200–7050	10–20

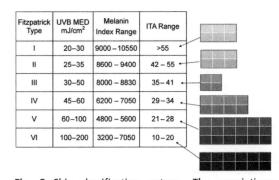

Fig. 3. Skin classification systems. The associations among skin classifications (ie, Fitzpatrick type, ITA) are shown along with corresponding melanin index ranges (spectroscopic assessment),[32] minimum erythema dose ranges,[33] and colors typified by each classification.[34] (*Data from* Refs.[32–34])

chambers.[43] Four conditions were evaluated: (1) dark-skinned keratinocytes with dark-skinned melanocytes (K_DM_D); (2) light keratinocytes with dark melanocytes (K_LM_D); (3) light keratinocytes (K_LM_L) with light melanocytes; and (4) dark keratinocytes with light melanocytes (K_DM_L). The grafted tissue skin color after healing was dark for K_DM_D and light for K_LM_L, as expected. The 2 mixed-origin tissues were intermediate in color but darker for K_LM_D than K_DM_L. For K_DM_D versus K_LM_D, melanin content (melanogenesis) was greater, although melanocyte density was comparable; melanosomes were more mature; and melanosomes were individually distributed in the basal and suprabasal keratinocytes, rather than in clusters. For K_DM_D versus K_LM_D, gene expression was greater for microohthalmia -associated transcription factor, tyrosinase, pmel-17, protein melan-A, endothelin-1, and proopiomelanocortin. Collectively, the findings indicate that keratinocytes controlled melanosome distribution. Although the experiment did not include cells from mixed white-African skin, a system that more accurately reflects skin color from a light and dark skin lineage, it nonetheless provides information about factors that affect skin color.

GENETICS: EVOLUTIONARY ASPECTS OF SKIN PIGMENTATION

Vitamin D, essential for bone mineralization, is produced in the skin with UV radiation, making sun exposure necessary for overall health. Evolutionary changes have included the loss of heavy coats of hair covering lightly pigmented skin. Hair loss and changes in thermoregulation were accompanied by increased naked skin pigmentation.[44] Genetic traits are known, generally, to show greater variability within local populations and lesser differences in main geographic areas, as exemplified in craniometrics.[45] However, the opposite result was found for skin color, wherein greater diversity occurred as a function of geography and, specifically, of the extent of UV exposure (latitude).[45]

Pigmentation characteristics changed after humans left Africa for more northern regions, such as Europe and east Asia.[46] The intensity of UV exposure lessens with distance from the equator and skin pigmentation decreased, presumably to facilitate sufficient UV interaction to produce vitamin D, and suggesting that pigmentation changes may be adaptive to manage the effects of UV exposure.[44]

UV exposure and vitamin D synthesis may be only part of the reason for skin color variation. The influence of ancestry on skin constitutive pigmentation, measured instrumentally as melanin index, was examined by admixture mapping of 34 to 36 ancestry-indicated genetic markers among African American, African Caribbean, Mexican, Hispanic, and Puerto Rican people. The correlations were moderate at best, with the highest for Puerto Rican people (0.66; range, 0.457–0.457) and high variability (correlation coefficients of −0.369 to 0.761) across groups.[47]

Genetic studies have identified at least 120 genes associated with human skin pigmentation but the melanocortin 1 receptor (MC1R) gene predominates in color-related skin differences/changes and was the first to be associated with normal skin variation.[12,48] It encodes the MC1R protein located on the surface of melanocytes and regulates the ratio of 2 melanin types, as well as other non–pigment-related functions.[49] The MC1R gene showed large allele variation (65 identified) in European populations but not in Asian or African groups[50] The findings over the last 15 years suggest that pigmentation diversity is a result of natural selection.[50]

ETHNIC SKIN: RESPONSE TO STRESS

The response to stress is essential in discussions about skin color, with the specific responses to the stress of UV radiation being a key feature of color classification systems. The skin mechanisms designed to modulate the damaging effects of UV radiation serve as surrogates for considering the effects of other stresses, such as laser treatments and topical products designed to correct various skin conditions.

Implications for Treatment

Skin treatments, such as the application of laser energy for smoothing wrinkles and skin whitening agents (eg, retinoic acid) for dark spots, may produce inflammation. Injury and resulting inflammation are potential adverse effects of scar treatment. Therefore, the impact of UV exposure on skin coloration (ie, the pigmentary response) is a useful model for considering the potential effects of other skin treatments. The influence of ethnicity/skin color is important clinically in deciding treatment of skin conditions, including scars, photodamage (eg, wrinkles, solar lentigines, hyperpigmentation), wounds, burns, and infections. Postinflammatory hyperpigmentation (PIH) in relation to skin color is reviewed next. The skin's response to UV radiation has been investigated extensively in relation to skin cancers and photoaging, thereby providing information relevant to the problem of PIH in scar development and treatment.

Hyperpigmentation occurs when the inflammatory source acts on prostaglandins

(PGE2, PGF2α), thromboxanes, and leukotrienes to stimulate tyrosinase, causing an increased synthesis of melanin and its transfer to keratinocytes and macrophages.[51] UVB exposure (350 nm) and postexposure pigmentation were explored in type III skin (n = 16) by treating skin sites with energies (n = 12) of 12 to 240 mJ/cm^2 and at 24 hours and 7 days for erythema index and melanin index versus untreated skin.[52] Erythema and melanin differences from control were not independent and change in melanin level was directly related to the intensity of inflammation (eg, energy level). Erythema and melanin differences were positively correlated, indicating more efficient melanin generation in darker skin. Studies across skin types (I–VI) or pigmentation levels are needed to fully establish the relationships among inflammation intensity, melanin response (ie, PIH), and inherent skin color.

Other patient characteristics may also contribute to the irritant response. For example, the atopic diathesis and the presence of a polymorphism on the tumor necrosis factor alpha gene at position 308 have individually and together been associated with increased susceptibility to skin irritants.[53–55] Consequently, patient experiences with skin care products provide insight regarding higher-than-expected response to treatments.

REFERENCES

1. Galdino GM, Vogel JE, Vander Kolk CA. Standardizing digital photography: it's not all in the eye of the beholder. Plast Reconstr Surg 2001;108: 1334–44.
2. Anderson RR, Parrish JA. The optics of human skin. J Invest Dermatol 1981;77:13–9.
3. Caspers PJ, Lucassen GW, Carter EA, et al. In vivo confocal Raman microspectroscopy of the skin: noninvasive determination of molecular concentration profiles. J Invest Dermatol 2001; 116:434–42.
4. Arce-Lopera C, Igarashi T, Nakao K, et al. Image statistics on the age perception of human skin. Skin Res Technol 2012;19(1):e273–8.
5. Hunt RWG. The reproduction of color. 6th edition. Chichester (United Kingdom): Wiley; 2004.
6. Wyszecki G, Stiles WS. Color science: concepts and methods, quantitative data and formulae. 2nd edition. New York: Wiley; 1982.
7. Chardon A, Cretois I, Hourseau C. Skin colour typology and suntanning pathways. Int J Cosmet Sci 1991;13:191–208.
8. Nordlund JJ, Boissy RE. The biology of melanocytes. In: Freinkel RK, Woodley DT, editors. The biology of the skin. New York: Parthenon Publishing Group; 2001. p. 113–31.
9. Morgan JE, Gilchrest B, Goldwyn RM. Skin pigmentation. Current concepts and relevance to plastic surgery. Plast Reconstr Surg 1975;56: 617–28.
10. Knudsen A, Brodersen R. Skin colour and bilirubin in neonates. Arch Dis Child 1989;64:605–9.
11. Takiwaki H. Measurement of skin color: practical application and theoretical considerations. J Med Invest 1998;44:121–6.
12. Brenner M, Hearing VJ. The protective role of melanin against UV damage in human skin. Photochem Photobiol 2008;84:539–49.
13. Rouzaud F, Kadekaro AL, Abdel-Malek ZA, et al. MC1R and the response of melanocytes to ultraviolet radiation. Mutat Res 2005;571:133–52.
14. Aubin F. Mechanisms involved in ultraviolet light-induced immunosuppression. Eur J Dermatol 2003; 13:515–23.
15. Kripke ML. Immunology and photocarcinogenesis. New light on an old problem. J Am Acad Dermatol 1986;14:149–55.
16. Fitzpatrick TB. The validity and practicality of sun-reactive skin types I through VI. Arch Dermatol 1988;124:869–71.
17. Weller R, Hunter J, Savin J, et al. Clinical dermatology. 4th edition. Malden (MA): Blackwell Publishing; 2008.
18. Sturm RA, Duffy DL, Box NF, et al. The role of melanocortin-1 receptor polymorphism in skin cancer risk phenotypes. Pigment Cell Res 2003;16:266–72.
19. Rhodes AR, Weinstock MA, Fitzpatrick TB, et al. Risk factors for cutaneous melanoma. A practical method of recognizing predisposed individuals. JAMA 1987; 258:3146–54.
20. Ravnbak MH. Objective determination of Fitzpatrick skin type. Dan Med Bull 2010;57:B4153.
21. He SY, McCulloch CE, Boscardin WJ, et al. Self-reported pigmentary phenotypes and race are significant but incomplete predictors of Fitzpatrick skin phototype in an ethnically diverse population. J Am Acad Dermatol 2014;71:731–7.
22. Ho BK, Robinson JK. Color bar tool for skin type self-identification: a cross-sectional study. J Am Acad Dermatol 2015;73:312–3.e1.
23. Kawai K, Kawai J, Nakagawa M, et al. Effects of detergents. In: Wilhelm K, Elsner P, Berardesca E, et al, editors. Bioengineering of the skin: skin surface imaging and analysis. Boca Raton (FL): CRC Press; 1997. p. 303–14.
24. Mattsson U, Jonsson A, Jontell M, et al. Digital image analysis (DIA) of colour changes in human skin exposed to standardized thermal injury and comparison with laser Doppler measurements. Comput Methods Programs Biomed 1996;50:31–42.
25. Coelho SG, Miller SA, Zmudzka BZ, et al. Quantification of UV-induced erythema and pigmentation

using computer-assisted digital image evaluation. Photochem Photobiol 2006;82:651–5.

26. Setaro M, Sparavigna A. Quantification of erythema using digital camera and computer-based colour image analysis: a multicentre study. Skin Res Technol 2002;8:84–8.

27. Colorimetry. CIE publications No. 15.2. In: Colorimetric illuminants (CIE S001); colorimetric observers (CIE S002). 2nd edition. Vienna (Austria): Central Bureau of the CIE; 1986.

28. Weatherall IL, Coombs BD. Skin color measurements in terms of CIELAB color space values. J Invest Dermatol 1992;99:468–73.

29. Alaluf S, Atkins D, Barrett K, et al. The impact of epidermal melanin on objective measurements of human skin colour. Pigment Cell Res 2002;15:119–26.

30. Del Bino S, Bernerd F. Variations in skin colour and the biological consequences of ultraviolet radiation exposure. Br J Dermatol 2013;169(Suppl 3):33–40.

31. Del Bino S, Sok J, Bessac E, et al. Relationship between skin response to ultraviolet exposure and skin color type. Pigment Cell Res 2006;19:606–14.

32. Eilers S, Bach DQ, Gaber R, et al. Accuracy of self-report in assessing Fitzpatrick skin phototypes I through VI. JAMA Dermatol 2013;149:1289–94.

33. Pathak MA, Fanselow DL. Photobiology of melanin pigmentation: dose/response of skin to sunlight and its contents. J Am Acad Dermatol 1983;9:724–33.

34. Saint-Leger D. The colour of the human skin: fruitful science, unsuitable wordings. Int J Cosmet Sci 2015;37:259–65.

35. Quevedo WC, Holstein TJ. General biology of mammalian pigmentation. In: Nordlund JJ, Boissy RE, Hearing VJ, et al, editors. The pigmentary system. Oxford (United Kingdom): Blackwell Publishing; 2006. p. 63–90.

36. Marks MS, Seabra MC. The melanosome: membrane dynamics in black and white. Nat Rev Mol Cell Biol 2001;2:738–48.

37. Costin GE, Hearing VJ. Human skin pigmentation: melanocytes modulate skin color in response to stress. FASEB J 2007;21:976–94.

38. Ito S, Wakamatsu K. Quantitative analysis of eumelanin and pheomelanin in humans, mice, and other animals: a comparative review. Pigment Cell Res 2003;16:523–31.

39. Valverde P, Healy E, Jackson I, et al. Variants of the melanocyte-stimulating hormone receptor gene are associated with red hair and fair skin in humans. Nat Genet 1995;11:328–30.

40. Chiarelli-Neto O, Ferreira AS, Martins WK, et al. Melanin photosensitization and the effect of visible light on epithelial cells. PLoS One 2014;9:e113266.

41. Alaluf S, Atkins D, Barrett K, et al. Ethnic variation in melanin content and composition in photoexposed and photoprotected human skin. Pigment Cell Res 2002;15:112–8.

42. Thong HY, Jee SH, Sun CC, et al. The patterns of melanosome distribution in keratinocytes of human skin as one determining factor of skin colour. Br J Dermatol 2003;149:498–505.

43. Yoshida Y, Hachiya A, Sriwiriyanont P, et al. Functional analysis of keratinocytes in skin color using a human skin substitute model composed of cells derived from different skin pigmentation types. FASEB J 2007;21:2829–39.

44. Jablonski NG, Chaplin G. The evolution of human skin coloration. J Hum Evol 2000;39:57–106.

45. Relethford JH. Apportionment of global human genetic diversity based on craniometrics and skin color. Am J Phys Anthropol 2002;118:393–8.

46. Hider JL, Gittelman RM, Shah T, et al. Exploring signatures of positive selection in pigmentation candidate genes in populations of East Asian ancestry. BMC Evol Biol 2013;13:150.

47. Parra EJ, Kittles RA, Shriver MD. Implications of correlations between skin color and genetic ancestry for biomedical research. Nat Genet 2004;36:S54–60.

48. Rees JL. Genetics of hair and skin color. Annu Rev Genet 2003;37:67–90.

49. Rees JL. The melanocortin 1 receptor (MC1R): more than just red hair. Pigment Cell Res 2000;13:135–40.

50. Rees JL, Harding RM. Understanding the evolution of human pigmentation: recent contributions from population genetics. J Invest Dermatol 2012;132:846–53.

51. Yamaguchi Y, Hearing VJ. Physiological factors that regulate skin pigmentation. Biofactors 2009;35:193–9.

52. Takiwaki H, Shirai S, Kohno H, et al. The degrees of UVB-induced erythema and pigmentation correlate linearly and are reduced in a parallel manner by topical anti-inflammatory agents. J Invest Dermatol 1994;103:642–6.

53. Allen MH, Wakelin SH, Holloway D, et al. Association of TNFA gene polymorphism at position -308 with susceptibility to irritant contact dermatitis. Immunogenetics 2000;51:201–5.

54. Davis JA, Visscher MO, Wickett RR, et al. Influence of tumour necrosis factor-alpha polymorphism-308 and atopy on irritant contact dermatitis in healthcare workers. Contact Dermatitis 2010;63:320–32.

55. de Jongh CM, John SM, Bruynzeel DP, et al. Cytokine gene polymorphisms and susceptibility to chronic irritant contact dermatitis. Contact Dermatitis 2008;58:269–77.

Index

Note: Page numbers of article titles are in **boldface** type.

Facial Plast Surg Clin N Am 25 (2017) 127–140
http://dx.doi.org/10.1016/S1064-7406(16)30128-6
1064-7406/17

Moving?

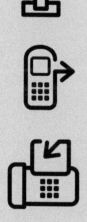

Printed and bound by CPI Group (UK) Ltd, Croydon, CR0 4YY

08/05/2025

01864696-0012